Earl Mindell, R.Ph., Ph.D.,

is also the author of

Earl Mindell's New Herb Bible

Earl Mindell's Supplement Bible

Earl Mindell's Secret Remedies

Earl Mindell's Anti-Aging Bible

Earl Mindell's Soy Miracle Cookbook

Earl Mindell's Soy Miracle

Earl Mindell's Food as Medicine

Earl Mindell's Vitamin Bible

EARL MINDELL'S
Peak Performance Bible

How to Look Great,
Feel Great, and Perform Better
in the Gym, at Work,
and in Bed

Earl Mindell, R.Ph., Ph.D.

A FIRESIDE BOOK
Published by Simon & Schuster
New York London Toronto Sydney Singapore

FIRESIDE
Rockefeller Center
1230 Avenue of the Americas
New York, NY 10020

Copyright © 2001 by Earl Mindell, R.Ph., Ph.D., and Carol Colman
All rights reserved,
including the right of reproduction
in whole or in part in any form.

FIRESIDE and colophon are registered trademarks
of Simon & Schuster, Inc.

Designed by Christine Weathersbee

Manufactured in the United States of America

10 9 8 7 6 5 4 3 2 1

Library of Congress Cataloging-in-Publication Data is available

ISBN 0-7432-0437-9

The ideas, procedures, and suggestions contained in this book are not intended to replace the services of a trained health professional. All matters regarding your health require medical supervision. You should consult a physician before adopting the procedures in this book. Any applications of the treatments set forth in this book are at the reader's discretion.

Acknowledgments

I wish to express my deep and lasting appreciation to the people who assisted me on this book, including J. Gabrielle Rabner, M.S., R.D., holistic nutritionist, for her help with the chapters on nutrition and teenage athletes. She's always a pleasure to work with! I would also like to thank Harold Segal, Ph.D.; Bernard Bubman, R.Ph.; Edward Powell, R.Ph.; Sal Messineo, Pharm.D.; Arnold Fox, M.D.; Dennis Huddleson, M.D.; Rory Jaffe, M.D.; Donald Cruden, O.D.; Nathan Sperling, D.D.S.; and Alan Kashin, R.Ph., Ph.D. A special thanks to Carol Colman; my editor, Caroline Sutton; and Nicole Diamond, assistant editor, for their help. Also, many thanks to my agent, Richard Curtis, for all his support through the years.

Contents

1

THE PEAK PERFORMANCE PHENOMENON

You're reading this book because you want to do everything better! You want to excel at the gym, win on the playing field, succeed at work or at school, and have energy to spare to enjoy your life. You're not alone. You're part of a growing trend of millions of men and women who are using performance enhancers: hundreds of new, cutting-edge supplements and meal-replacement products that can help you look and feel better. Some performance supplements build muscle, burn fat, and boost athletic performance. Others heighten energy and stamina, speed recovery after a workout, or boost sexual function. Still others enhance focus and mental alertness. These products are fast becoming best-sellers among weekend athletes, dieters, baby boomers who feel they are losing their edge, and, even, teenage athletes. In the United States alone, consumers are spending *billions* of dollars on performance supplements.

I am writing this book to help you choose the performance supplements that will best suit your needs. There's a great deal of hype surrounding performance supplements. Flip through the pages of any fitness magazine or turn on TV, and you will see advertisements touting the benefits of these high-tech wonders. *Burn fat! Get ripped! Rev up your sex life! Get energized!* They all sound great, but do all they work? Some really do live up to the hype, and you will learn about them in this book. But not all performance supplements are created equal. Many are safe and effective, but others are worthless and downright *unsafe*, particularly for teenagers. Still others are old supplements in new bottles; that is, supplements that have been around for years, but are now repackaged and given hot new names to cash in on this trend. I don't mean to disparage these old supplements—many of them are some of the best performance products on the market. To my way of thinking, however, it's not fair to let consumers believe that they are new (and often, charge more for them).

How do you distinguish between good products and bad products? First, high-quality products are usually backed by good research, that is, some scientific studies confirming their safety and efficacy. Second, there should be ample anecdotal support for products. In other words, if a product is supposed to help people build muscle or lose weight, there ought to be hordes of happy consumers willing to tell their stories. By the time you have finished this book, you will know which peak performance supplements truly live up to their name, and which are a waste of money.

As many of you may know, I've been writing about supplements for more than twenty years. I am a pharmacist and a master herbalist. Published in 1979, *Earl Mindell's Vitamin Bible* is still widely read today, and is generally regarded as one of the books that helped popularize vitamins throughout the world. Nearly a decade ago, I wrote *Earl Mindell's Herb Bible*, which helped bring herbal medicine to millions of homes. When I first wrote the *Herb Bible*, few people had even heard of herbs such as echinacea, ginseng, and ginkgo biloba, which are now household names. Today, one-third of all Americans use herbal supplements and related products. (In fact, there are so many new herbal products that an updated edition of the *Herb Bible* was published in 2000.) *The Peak Performance Bible* has a similar mission to that of the *Vitamin Bible* and the *Herb Bible*. This book is written for the both the new and experienced user of performance products. Similarly, I am confident that many of the worthy peak performance products that I introduce in this book will be around in decades to come.

What Are Peak Performance Supplements?

Peak performance supplements consist of a wide variety of seemingly un-related supplements with one thing in common—they are designed to enhance your body or your mind. This diverse group of supplements include vitamins, minerals, herbs, protein powders, amino acids, en-zymes, hormones, sports drinks, and sports bars. (If you are unfamiliar with some of these terms, check the section at the end of this chapter, "Answers to Commonly Asked Questions.") They are sold over the counter at natural food stores, discount pharmacies, general merchan-dise stores, supermarkets and even on the Internet.

Peak performance supplements come in many different forms: pills, capsules, tablets, powders that can be mixed with water or juice, beverages, extracts, food bars, and in lotions and gels that can be ap-plied topically. Choose the form that is easiest for you to use. For exam-ple, if you hate to swallow pills, you may be able to use a liquid or extract. In some cases, I do recommend one particular form of a supple-ment because I feel that it is the most effective, or least likely to produce unwanted side effects. After I describe a product, I tell you how to use it. Please follow my directions, and be careful not to exceed my recom-mended dose. Although most performance products are safe at even high doses, some can cause adverse side effects (like stomach upset) at higher-than-recommended doses.

How to Buy Peak Performance Supplements

You walk into a natural food store or a discount pharmacy, and you see row upon row of supplements. How do you choose the right brands? Nutritional supplements are not regulated by the government so, to be sure that you are getting the best-quality products, stick to brands from reputable, well-known manufacturers that take special steps to ensure safety and effectiveness. Some unscrupulous manufacturers may water down a product so that it does not contain the quantity of supplement that it should. This is unfortunate, and has hurt the reputation of the entire industry. Most of the well-known manufacturers, however, do have good quality control. Here are some tips as to how to choose the best products:

- Buy products that come in tamperproof packages with both an inside and outside seal.
- Look for products that state on the label that they are laboratory tested and guaranteed, which means that the product has been assayed by an independent laboratory.
- To be sure the product is fresh, look for an expiration date on the package; an old supplement may have lost some of its effectiveness.
- Look for a quality-control number on the package. If something is wrong, the manufacturer can quickly pull the product off the shelf.

Just a reminder: Most supplements don't come in childproof packages. If there are children in your home, be sure to put your supplements in a childproof container, or be scrupulous about keeping them out of reach of children.

How to Take
Peak Performance Supplements

Unless otherwise noted, take your supplements with a full glass of water, after eating, to enhance absorption. There are times, however, that I will tell you to take a particular supplement before meals on an empty stomach. It's usually best to take your supplements in two doses: one in the morning and one in the afternoon. In all likelihood, you will need to carry your supplements with you to work so that you don't miss a midday dose. I recommend that you take a few minutes on a weekend to set up your week's supply of prepackaged supplements in plastic baggies or special pill containers. Take one bag of supplements in the morning, and take another bag to work. This way, you won't have to count pills every day, and you'll have your supplements at your fingertips when you need them.

Some performance supplements are best taken up to an hour before exercise to boost stamina and energy, or immediately following exercise to speed up recovery, which means that you'll need to bring your supplements with you to the gym or playing field.

Some supplements can be taken daily like vitamin pills, others should be taken only occasionally to get a desired result, or should be used only for a limited time. If a supplement works well, why not take it every day? First, overusing some supplements can render them ineffective. You'll be wasting your money! Second, some supplements may be not be safe for long-term use. So, please follow my directions carefully.

Some supplements can be taken with prescription drugs, other should not. When in doubt about taking a supplement, check with your pharmacist, physician, or natural healer. They will be able to tell you about potential interactions between your medication and your supplements.

At times, I don't recommend a precise dose for a particular supplement; rather, I will give a range of doses. Some people are highly susceptible to the effects of medications of any kind and may only require a small dose of a particular substance to get an effect. Older adults tend to fall in this category. To make sure that a supplement agrees with you, start with the smaller dose and work your way up to the maximum dose.

Use your common sense. Don't take a stimulating supplement at night when you want to sleep, or a supplement that promotes sleep when you need to feel energized and active. Be especially careful not to use natural tranquilizers or sleep aids if you have to drive a car or operate heavy machinery (and that includes the machines at the gym).

Supplements are sold separately, or in multicombination formulas. When you take more than one supplement, the peak performance term is *stacking*. In some cases, the multicombination supplement is more economical than buying several different ones. However, in some cases, the doses for each supplement could be so low that the product is a waste of money. If you chose to use multicombination supplements, read the label carefully to make sure that you are getting the full dose that I recommend. Also be sure that you're not getting any ingredient that you don't want.

Store your supplements in a cool, dry place out of direct sunlight. Some supplements need to be refrigerated; read the label for precise instructions.

How to Use This Book

At the core of this book is chapter 2, "The Hot Hundred Peak Performance Supplements." These include some new, exciting, cutting-edge supplements, as well as some old favorites that have new applications or were the subject of new studies that either confirm or negate manufacturers' claims. Rest assured, I don't take 100 supplements a day, and I don't expect you to either! Read the Hot Hundred to decide which, if any, of these supplements can help you achieve your goals.

Chapters 3 through 10 can help you better refine your choice of supplements. These chapters deal with specific topics (like the best supplements for energy and stamina, how to improve your brain power, and how to enhance your sex life), and can better show you how to incorporate the right supplements into your life.

The *Peak Performance Bible* is written for people of all ages and all levels of strength. I have included important information for body builders who want to get bigger, overweight folks who want to get leaner, and weekend athletes who are desperately trying to stay fit. Because I am concerned about such problems as steroid abuse and eating disorders among high-school students, I have devoted a chapter to teenagers. Because I am equally concerned about out-of-shape adults, I have also written a chapter called "Peak Performance Forever! The Midlife Tuneup."

I don't want to suggest that any pill or potion can make you healthy and strong. Throughout this book, I place equal importance on nutrition, exercise, and a sensible lifestyle. Don't believe manufacturers that promise you can have the body of your dreams simply by using their product. These claims are exaggerations, at best, and outright lies, at worst.

Answers to Commonly Asked Questions

Here are some answers to commonly asked questions about supplements in general and peak performance products in particular.

What are vitamins and minerals?

Vitamins are organic substances that are essential for life but usually not produced by the body. Therefore, you must get vitamins from your food or vitamin supplements. Most vitamins are measured in grams, mcg. (1/1,000,000 gram), or mg. (1/1000 gram). There is one exception: Fat soluble vitamins (A,D,E, K) are measured in IU (international units). The rule of thumb is 1 IU=1mg.

Minerals are natural substances that are found throughout the body that must also be obtained through food or supplements. No minerals are made by your body. Minerals are essential for normal cell function, teeth, bones, and connective tissue. There are two types of minerals: essential minerals and trace minerals. Essential minerals need to be consumed in greater volume and are measured in mg. or grams. We require only a minuscule amount of trace minerals; they are measured in mcg.

Why do you often recommend doses of vitamins and minerals that are higher than the Daily Values?

The Daily Values (formerly called RDAs) are the U.S. government's determinations of the bare minimum of vitamins and minerals needed each day to prevent a deficiency disease like *scurvy* (a severe lack of vitamin C) or *beri beri* (a severe lack of vitamin B1.) Most of us don't think about these diseases anymore because they are rare in the western world. The problem with the DVs is that they don't reflect what we need to enjoy optimal health and vitality. When the DVs were first designed, we knew very little about how our cells worked and how vitamins and minerals function in our bodies. Today, we know that vitamins and minerals can play a role in preventing disease, including heart disease, cancer, and depression. The doses of vitamins and minerals I recommend are based on studies reflect that reflect this new way of thinking.

You may notice that I also recommend many supplements that are not in the DVs, including essential fatty acids or *carotenoids* (compounds found in plants.) Although a lack of these substances does not cause a known deficiency disease, they are critical for good health and, therefore, I believe, are as important as supplements in the DVs.

Do I need to take supplements if I eat a well-balanced diet?

Most Americans don't eat as well as they think they do. Numerous studies have shown that, on any given day, most Americans are deficient in one or more of the vitamins and minerals listed in the Daily Values. Only a handful of people actually consume the five to eight servings of fruits and vegetables daily recommended by the National Cancer Institute. I pride myself on being a careful eater, yet, I know that it's extremely difficult to get all the nutrients I need from my food alone. For one thing, the vitamin and mineral content in fruits and vegetables vary according to growing conditions; therefore, the nutrient content is unpredictable. In some cases, it's impossible to get enough of a particular vitamin from food alone. For example, in order to get my recommended 400IUs daily of vitamin E, you would have to eat close to 100 pounds of broiled liver or 125 teaspoons of peanut oil. Isn't it easier to simply take a supplement?

What's an herb?

Herb refers to any plant or part of a plant (leaf, root, bark, seeds, or extract) used for medicine or cooking. Plants have been used in the prevention and treatment of illness for thousands of years. Plants are a rich source of *phytochemicals*, natural substances that are pharmacologically active; that is, they exert a profound effect on certain animal tissues and organs. In fact, it may surprise you to learn that up to half of all prescription drugs are derived from plants, including *digitalis* (from the foxglove plant), *aspirin* (from the bark of the white willow tree), and *quinine* (from the bark of the cinchona tree). In fact, several of the hottest peak performance supplements are actually herbs.

What are muscle builders?

A *muscle builder* is any substance that has *anabolic action*, which means it helps build or maintain lean tissue. Many substances purport to be muscle builders, but only a few actually deliver the goods. Contrary to what some manufacturers may suggest, there is no supplement on the planet that can build significant muscle mass without exercise.

What are thermogenic agents?

Thermogenic agents are supplements that turn up your metabolism, resulting in the burning of more fat. These supplements tend to be stimulants, and can have some unpleasant side effects (like heart palpitations and jitteriness.) If used judiciously, along with a sensible eating plan and exercise, they may help enhance weight loss. They are not for everyone, and I believe they should be used under the supervision of a physician or natural healer.

What's a recovery product?

Vigorous exercise depletes your body of important nutrients and energy. *Recovery products* help you bounce back faster, and can enhance the effect of your workout. Recovery products are not necessary for everybody—they are most useful for serious athletes who work out hard at least three times a week.

What are hormones and prohormones?

Hormones are chemical messengers in the body that tell our cells what to do. They regulate virtually every body function, from sexual growth and development, to how we think, to the beating of our hearts. The male hormone *testosterone* is instrumental in making and maintaining muscle. *Prohormones* (like DHEA) are precursors to the production of other hormones.

Can women and men use the same peak performance products?

Most of the products mentioned in this book are fine for both women and men, with some exceptions. In particular, I do not recommend that women use any products that boost male hormones because they could have undesirable side effects.

What are enzymes and co-enzymes?

An *enzyme* is a protein found in living cells that brings about a chemical change. A *co-enzyme* works with an enzyme to produce a particular reaction.

What does cycling mean?

Cycling means periodically changing your workout or supplement regimen. Many athletes believe that their bodies quickly become accustomed to a particular regimen, reducing its initial impact. Therefore, switching regimens may help accrue maximum benefits.

2

THE HOT
HUNDRED

There are hundreds of peak performance products on the market, with more being introduced each day. In this chapter, I have narrowed the number down to the Hot Hundred, the supplements that I feel you need to know about. Although I recommend most of these supplements wholeheartedly, I have reservations about a few others. I will tell you when I don't think a supplement is worth the risk, or if it's not suitable for people with specific problems. My purpose is to provide you with enough information so that you can make the right choice for yourself.

When it comes to supplements, I am biased in favor of those that promote overall health in addition to enhancing mental and physical performance. As you read through the Hot Hundred, you may be surprised to see how many of these supplements are actually good for you! In addition to improving strength, stamina, and endurance, many also protect against heart disease, cancer, arthritis, and other chronic ailments often associated with aging. Use them in good health!

Some people need to be extra careful about using supplements. Pregnant or nursing women, teenagers, people with chronic health conditions, or those taking prescription medications should check with their physicians or natural healers before taking any medication or supplement.

Hot hundred entries that appear in entries other than their own are designated by an asterisk.

Hot Hundred

1. Alanine
2. Androstenedione
3. Antioxidants
4. Arctic Root
5. Arginine
6. Arnica
7. Ashwagandha
8. Aspirin
9. Astaxanthin
10. Bee Pollen
11. Beta Sitosterol
12. Boswellia
13. Branched-Chain Amino Acids
14. Caffeine
15. Calcium
16. Carnitine
17. Carotenoids
18. Cayenne
19. Chondroitin
20. Chromium
21. Chrysin
22. Ciwujia
23. CLA
24. Colostrum
25. CO-Q10
26. Cordyceps
27. Creatine
28. DHA
29. DHEA
30. DHT Blockers
31. DIM
32. Natural Diuretics
33. DMAE
34. Ephedra
35. Essential Fatty Acids
36. Estrogen Blockers
37. Fat Blockers
38. Flavonoids
39. Forskolin
40. Gamma Oryzanol
41. Ginkgo
42. Ginseng
43. Glucomannan
44. Glucosamine
45. Glutamine
46. Glutathione
47. Glycerol
48. Green Tea
49. Guarana
50. Guggul
51. HMB
52. Homeopathic Growth Factors
53. Horny Goat Weed
54. Human Growth Hormone Releasing Agents
55. Hydroxycitric Acid

56. Ipriflavone
57. Iron
58. 7-Keto
59. Leucine
60. Lipoic Acid
61. MACA
62. Magnesium
63. Methionine
64. MSM
65. NAC
66. NADH
67. OKG
68. Ornithine
69. Panthothenic Acid
70. Pheromones
71. Phosphatidlyserine
72. Potassium
73. Proanthocyanidins
74. Pyruvate
75. Reishi Mushroom
76. Rhododendron
    Caucasicum
77. Ribose
78. SAM-e
79. Selenium
80. Sodium
81. Soy Protein
82. Sports Bars
83. Sports Drinks
84. Synephrine
85. T-Boosters
86. TMG
87. Tribulus
88. Tyrosine
89. Vanadium
90. Velvet Deer Antler
91. Vinpocetine
92. Vitamin B-1
93. Vitamin C
94. Vitamin E
95. Water
96. Whey Protein Powder
97. White Willow
98. Yohimbe
99. Zinc
100. ZMA

ALANINE

Alanine is a nonessential amino acid, a building block of protein. *Nonessential* doesn't mean it's not important; it means that the body can produce it on its own and, theoretically, doesn't need to obtain it from food. If you work out hard, however, you may require more alanine than your body can make on its own. Alanine is included in many products designed for body builders, such as whey protein powder and amino acids, for good reason—it's a major component of connective tissue. Anyone who engages in weightlifting or endurance sports is putting incredible pressure on their joints, and must take special precaution to protect their precious cartilage. If you don't take care of your joints, you run the risk of developing premature arthritis. Alanine, along with other joint-sparing supplements, could help prevent serious joint problems down the road.

Alanine is also involved in *glucose alanine cycle*, which provides energy to muscles, and may promote muscle growth. In fact, when you work out hard, you rapidly break down alanine, which means you are using up your supply.

Alanine is not just a muscle builder: It offers special health benefits to men. A study published in the *Journal of American Geriatrics* reported that alanine supplementation (along with glycine and glutamic acid) reduced the symptoms of enlarged prostate, a common problem of men over forty. I mention this because so many of the testosterone-boosting performance supplements (T-boosters) can do just the opposite—they may promote prostate growth, and are not suitable for men with prostate problems.

Possible Benefits

May help prevent wearing down of cartilage.
Muscle builder.
Protects prostate.

How to Use It

Take 500–3000 mg. daily, between meals.

ANDROSTENEDIONE (ANDRO)

facts *Androstenedione* or *andro* is a hormone produced by the body as part of the production pathway for testosterone. (It is also the same pathway used to make the female hormone, estrogen.) It may surprise you to learn that both men and women produce testosterone and estrogen, but men produce more testosterone, and women produce more estrogen. In the body, andro is made from two other well-known hormones, pregnenolone and DHEA. When taken as a supplement, andro may temporarily boost testosterone levels, which is supposed to help build muscle and enhance endurance.

Once an obscure supplement used primarily by body builders looking for an alternative to anabolic steroids, andro went mainstream in 1998, when Mark McGwire admitted using the stuff during his record seventy-home-run year. Overnight, sales of andro increased 500 percent. Since then, andro has been a lightning rod for controversy. Some critics contend that it is unsafe, others say it is ineffective, and still others say it is no different from potent anabolic steroids, and should not be sold over the counter. Andro has been banned by the Olympics, the NCAA, the NFL, men and women's tennis tours, and, most recently, by the NBA. As a result of all this negative publicity, andro sales are on the decline.

When it comes to andro, there are more questions than answers. Does it really work? Is it dangerous? Does it offer the benefits of anabolic steroids without the risks? Many body builders and many professional athletes believe that andro has made them bigger and better, but scientific studies of andro are scarce and inconsistent. One oft-cited study, performed in 1962 on four nonathletic women, showed that 100 mg. andro taken orally can boost testosterone levels. In the 1980s, East German athletes were given andro in the form of a nasal spray, which also reportedly raised testosterone levels. When andro became popular in the West, a handful of studies sponsored by manufacturers showed that andro spiked testosterone levels in male body builders. However, none of these studies correlated andro use with increased muscle mass or improved performance. In 1999, the *Journal of the American Medical Association* reported on a study comparing testosterone levels in twenty young men who were on a moderate, eight-week weight-training program. Half the men were given 300 mg. of andro daily; the other half received a placebo. At the end of eight weeks, the researchers found no difference in either muscle strength or mass in the men taking andro *versus* the placebo. What they did find was that the men taking andro had higher levels of *estrogen* than the placebo takers. This raised a red flag—high levels of estrogen in men have been associated with heart disease, *gynecomstia* (breast enlargement), and an increased risk of some forms of cancer. Still another study raised concerns that andro could make men more violent and aggressive, similar to the effect of anabolic steroids.

Within andro, there are different products with slight variations in chemical structures. Manufacturers make a big deal about these differences, although studies are scarce. For example, 4-Andriol (4-androstenediol) is reputed to be a very potent T-booster and is quite pricey. Nor-Androstenedione (nor-adione) is supposed to keep estrogen in check, and grow bigger muscles. Nor-4-Androstenediol (nor-4-adiol) is supposed to be a powerful muscle enhancer, but low on libido boosting.

As far as I'm concerned, there's not enough evidence confirming that any form of andro works well enough to offset the potential risks. Although studies have shown that testosterone supplementation can build muscle and increase strength, there is absolutely no evidence that andro does the same thing, and compelling evidence that it may not. I am adamant that teenagers and women should avoid it. Teenage boys make enough testosterone on their own, in fact, taking a testosterone-boosting supplement may suppress their own testosterone production. This could have long-term negative effects on their growth and development. Women should not take a testosterone-boosting product unless it is under the supervision of a physician. Hormones are unpredictable; you need just the right dose or the side effects can be unpleasant (hair where you don't want it) and downright dangerous (like cancer).

If a grown man chooses to use andro, he must do so understanding there are potential risks. We don't know the short term of effect of boosting testosterone. Some physicians worry that andro could promote the growth of prostate tumors. If exposed to a potent hormone, a tumor that might have lain dormant for years could suddenly start to grow. If you do use andro, be sure to have your PSA levels (*prostate-specific antigen*, a marker for prostate cancer) checked by your physician and to have a digital prostate examination annually. Also, keep an eye on your cholesterol levels. Andro can lower HDL, or good cholesterol, which protects against heart disease. If you see a negative change in your blood lipid levels, I strongly recommend that you discontinue using andro.

Potential Benefits

Reputed to boost testosterone.

Enhances muscle growth.

How to Use It

If you're using an andro product (or any other T-booster) you should do so under the supervision of a knowledgeable doctor or natural healer. You should have your hormone levels monitored to be sure that you are staying within normal range. In addition, be vigilant about monitoring your prostate for problems.

ANTIOXIDANTS

You've probably heard that antioxidants are good for your health and may help prevent cancer, heart disease, diabetes, cataracts, arthritis, and Alzheimer's disease. What you may not know is that antioxidants are of special importance for athletes and body builders. In fact, the harder you work out, the more you need antioxidant protection.

Antioxidants are a family of vitamins, minerals, and other nutrients that occur naturally in many foods, and are also produced by the body. They include vitamins C and E, lipoic acid, and co-enzyme Q10. They protect us against damage caused by *free radicals*, unstable oxygen molecules that can harm healthy cells, even turning them cancerous. Free radicals are produced by the body as a natural byproduct of energy production. Chemicals found in the environment, including toxins in food, pesticides, smoke, pollutants, and even the sun's UV rays can trigger the production of free radicals in the body.

As we know, exercise does wonderful things for your body and your mind—it strengthens your muscles, builds bone, and boosts mood. It makes you look great and feel great. *Aerobic exercise* in particular (the kind that increases lung capacity and oxygen consumption) has long been touted as being protective against heart disease. Recent studies suggest, however, that intense aerobic exercise, performed over a long period of time, may have some undesirable side effects. Here's why: When you work out hard, your body requires more energy. In order to meet those energy needs, you need to take in more oxygen. In fact, oxygen uptake during intense aerobic exercise can increase by ten to fifteen fold! The problem is that, the more oxygen you burn, the more free radicals you make, quickly depleting your body's natural supply of antioxidants. This could have serious consequences down the road. Numerous animal studies have documented that, after vigorous exercise, endurance-trained animals showed a marked decline in key antioxidants and signs of injury to muscle-cell membranes. It's not just endurance-trained animals at risk, people are, too. Ironically, those who appear to be most fit may be at greatest risk. For example, marathon runners frequently succumb to respiratory infections after the competition, a phenomenon that used to puzzle researchers. Today, we know that the vulnerability is due to a decline in antioxidants, which impairs immune function. If you are an endurance athlete, the antidote is to get enough antioxidants in your diet and to take the right antioxidant supplements to compensate for your increased free radical load. A diet rich in antioxidant foods (see "Peak Performance Nutrition") can help stem the damage, but so can taking antioxidant supplements.

Possible Benefits

Help promote recovery after work out.

Help prevent degenerative diseases associated with aging.

How to Use It

I take a formula that has 30 antioxidants including C, E, selenium, alpha lipoic acid, green tea, grape-seed extract, glutathione, and NAC. Antioxidants are *synergistic*, which means that they work better when combined with each other.

ARCTIC ROOT

 Although new to the United States, *arctic root* has been used for hundreds of years in Asia and Russia. Known as arctic root, or *Rhodiola rosea*, this herb fortifies us against stress, increases energy and stamina, and enhances the fat-burning effect of exercise. Arctic root is a member of the *Crassulaceae* family of plants, native to the arctic regions of eastern Siberia. During the Cold War, the Russians kept research about arctic root under wraps, allegedly to give their athletes an advantage in international competitions. Arctic root is an *adaptogen*, that is, a compound derived from plants that can help mediate the effects of environmental stress on the body. Known in Europe as the *ginseng alternative*, arctic root has all the energizing benefits of ginseng without causing the jitteriness that ginseng often does. It is also completely nontoxic, even at high doses. So, why do body builders and athletes need arctic root? Although exercise offers many benefits, intense exercise can be very stressful physically. When we are under physical or mental stress, our bodies produce a hormone called *cortisol*, which helps the body cope with the immediate stress, but has some nasty side effects. In particular, high levels of cortisol put the body in a *catabolic state*, in which protein is broken for energy, which tears down muscle—precisely the last thing a body builder wants! Arctic root has been shown to counteract the negative effects of cortisol, which makes body builders happy for obvious reasons, but controlling cortisol is important for other reasons, too. Cortisol overload can increase the risk of many diseases, including heart disease, cancer, diabetes, Alzheimer's disease, and osteoporosis. Cortisol not only hurts us on the inside, it hurts us on the outside. Cortisol makes our bodies retain fat, especially around our middle. If your once slim physique is becoming apple-shaped, blame it on cortisol!

Keeping cortisol under wraps is not all that arctic root does: It normalizes levels of serotonin and epinephrine, important brain chemicals involved in mood. Some people find that it is also effective for mild depression.

Researchers at Georgian State Hospital studied arctic root's effect on weight loss and fat metabolism. In a study involving seventy men and sixty women, researchers gave 300 mg. of arctic root to obese patients daily, for ninety days. The patients were put on a healthy diet and told to take a thirty to forty minute walk after each meal. Another group of obese patients was put on the same diet and walking regimen without the arctic root. At the end of study, the patients taking arctic root lost on average, 11 percent of their body weight. Those not taking arctic root lost only 4 percent. The right diet and exercise can help you lose weight, but it happens a lot faster when you take arctic root!

Arctic root is so highly prized in Russia that it was given to Russian cosmonauts to help them deal with the enormously stressful effects of space travel, and was one of the few plants selected by the Russian space agency to be cultivated in space. Arctic root has gained fame in Europe as the herb of choice for several popular soccer teams. Russian scientists claim that arctic root has many of the beneficial effects of anabolic steroids in terms of promoting better performance, but none of the negative side effects. Indeed, numerous studies, all performed in Russia, attest to arctic root's effectiveness.

Possible Benefits

Enhances physical endurance.
Relieves stress.
Promotes feelings of well-being.
Improves muscle-to-fat ratio.

How to Use It

Take one 100 mg. capsule daily, before breakfast, on an empty stomach.

For high-stress days, take one 100 mg. before breakfast and one 100 mg. before lunch.

Some people may find arctic root stimulating; do not take it too close to bedtime.

ARGININE

Arginine is an *amino acid*, a building block of protein. It **facts** may also be the building block for better muscles and a better sex life. Arginine can increase the body's production of *nitric oxide*, a gas that the body needs to dilate blood vessels, which improves blood flow throughout the body. What does this have to do with sex? Everything! Good blood flow to the penis is essential for achieving and maintaining a strong erection. That's why men with circulatory problems, like atherosclerosis, have problems getting and keeping an erection. In addition to anecdotal reports from happy users, several studies have found that arginine supplementation can enhance male sexual performance. Does arginine work as well for women? It would make sense that anything that improves blood flow to the pelvis would also increase sexual pleasure in women, but it's never been studied.

Natural healers prescribe arginine for men with low sperm count; it helps boost sperm count and motility in some, but not all, men.

When combined with the amino acid ornithine, arginine can boost production of growth hormone, important to grow muscles and lose fat. As we age, levels of growth hormone decline, leaving us fatter and flabbier. When combined with exercise, arginine may help retain lean body mass in older people; it appears to increase the body's production of creatine.

Arginine is used in hospitals to accelerate wound healing in older people who do not mend as quickly as young people. It also lowers cholesterol, which makes it heart healthy. New research shows that arginine helps to enhance brain function in dementia cases.

Very high doses of arginine—well beyond what I recommend—may stimulate the growth of tumors. Animal studies have not been consistent: Some show that high doses of arginine can grow tumors, others show that it thwarts their growth. Remember, arginine increases growth hormone, which is good, because it stimulates cell repair and production of new cells, but it could also stimulate a tumor to grow faster. At the same time, however, it boosts immune function, which gives the body ammunition to fight cancer. To be on the safe side, stick to my recommended doses.

Do not use arginine if you have kidney or liver disease, unless under your doctor's supervision. Avoid arginine if you have either genital or oral herpes; it can stimulate replication of the virus, unless you are taking the time-released form.

Your body makes arginine. It is also found in dairy, meat, fish, nuts, and poultry.

Possible Benefits

Harder, stronger erections.
May help increase sperm count in infertile men.
Promotes healing of wounds.

How to Use It

Take up to two 1500 mg. time-released arginine twice daily, with or without food. (I do—I call it sex in a bottle!)

ARNICA

facts Here's a peak performance supplement that's great for both serious athletes and weekend warriors. *Arnica* is a homeopathic remedy for overworked, sore muscles and minor strains and sprains. It's sold in spray or gel form to be used directly on the injured area (I always keep a tube of arnica gel in my medicine chest) or can be taken orally, but only in homeopathic doses. In full potency, arnica can be poisonous. For those of you unfamiliar with homeopathy, let me fill you in. It may sound a bit odd, but homeopathic preparations are very dilute forms of substances that, if taken in large doses, can create the symptoms you are trying to treat! The potency of the homeopathic substance is in inverse proportion to its dilution. So, for example, I recommend an oral form of arnica that is arnica 6c, which means it is diluted to $10,000 \times 6$. Interestingly, the more dilute a homeopathic substance, the greater its strength! Okay, so this may not make a lot of intuitive sense. Suffice it to say that prestigious medical journals like *Lancet* and the *British Medical Journal* have confirmed that homeopathic remedies are effective for certain conditions. In fact, in Britain, the royal family is treated by a homeopathic physician along with a conventional physician. All I can tell you is that arnica seems to work.

Of course, there's a time to self-medicate, and a time to get medical advice. If you have a strain or sprain that is very painful, swells up badly, or doesn't get better within a few days, do see your doctor.

Possible Benefits

Relieves post-workout pain.

May help heal sprain, strains, and sore muscles.

Helps eliminate black-and-blue marks after plastic surgery.

How to Use It

Externally: Massage gel or use spray directly on affected area. Don't apply arnica to broken skin.

Internally: Use homeopathic-strength arnica only (arnica 6c). Follow the directions on the package. If you are very sore after working out, try taking arnica before and after your workout. It doesn't work for everybody but, then again, neither does aspirin or ibuprofen.

· ·

ASHWAGANDHA

· ·

We in the West like to believe that we invented performance supplements, and that we are the very definition of *cutting edge*. In reality, when we compare ourselves to other cultures, we fall behind the curve. For thousands of years, traditional healers have been using natural substances to increase strength and stamina. Today, a new generation of fitness buffs are rediscovering the wisdom of the ancients.

In recent years, there has been an explosion of interest in *Ayurvedic medicine*, the traditional healing practices of India. *Ayurvedic*, which literally means knowledge of life, dates back to 1000 B.C. Today, we use the term *integrative* medicine to describe physicians who combine conventional medicine with alternative remedies, nutrition, and spiritual healing. The Ayurvedic system of medicine does all that and more. Unlike Western medicine, which emphasizes treating illness, Ayurvedic practitioners are equally concerned with maintaining health and vitality. The Ayurvedic pharmacy contains many tonic herbs that are not only used during times of illnesses, but are prescribed to keep you functioning at peak capacity. *Ashwagandha*, often called *Indian ginseng*, is an herb that is known for its ability to increase energy, sexual vigor, and stamina. In animal studies, ashwagandha has been shown to increase weight and muscle development, and improve memory in aging animals. Although there are no clinical studies to date that have shown that ashwagandha does the same in humans, there are numerous anecdotal reports. Since ashwagandha has been used as a tonic herb for thousands of years, I believe that there is a strong basis for these claims.

Ayurvedic healers boast that ashwagandha is better than ginseng; they cite studies showing that animals given ashwagandha can swim for longer periods of time than those given ginseng. They also contend that, unlike some forms of ginseng, ashwagandha does not make you feel edgy or shaky, and does not cause insomnia. In fact, it's been used to treat stress-related conditions.

Steroidlike compounds known as *withanolides* are believed to be the active ingredient in ashwagandha.

Who will benefit the most from ashwagandha? I believe that ashwagandha is not necessarily for the very young, but is a wonderful performance supplement for people forty plus. In addition to increasing energy, it offers a wide range of anti-aging benefits. For example, ashwagandha also boosts immune function, which declines as we age. It is also a natural anti-inflammatory, and has been used as a treatment for joint inflammation and arthritis. If you are beginning to feel that you are losing some of your zest, this is one supplement that you should consider taking.

Possible Benefits

Enhances energy and mood.

Relieves joint pain.

Boosts immune function.

How to Use It

Take up to three 4.5 mg. tablets daily.

• •

ASPIRIN

• •

facts Good old aspirin! It's been around for more than a century and, every decade or so, it manages to reinvent itself. In the twentieth century, aspirin was primarily used as a painkiller. Today, aspirin is hotter than ever as part of the *ECA stack* (ephedrine, caffeine, aspirin), the fat burner of choice at gyms and health clubs around the country. Aspirin is a synthetic version of *salicin*, a natural derivative of the bark of the white willow tree, which is sometimes used instead of aspirin in the ECA stack. Some studies have shown that aspirin has a synergistic effect with ephedra, which means that aspirin enhances ephedra's fat-burning potential. The ECA combination turns up metabolism, which produces more weight loss than can be achieved through dieting alone. (See page 72.) The ECA stack appears to spare lean muscle tissue, which is especially important to dieters and body builders striving for single-digit body-fat perfection.

There's a reason people take aspirin for their aches and pains. Aspirin is an anti-inflammatory. It works the same way as other non-steroidal anti-inflammatories (NSAIDs). It blocks the formation of *prostaglandins*, hormonelike substances in the body that can trigger an inflammatory response. Inflammation is what makes you hurt after your workout. Inflammation can also damage healthy cells, and has been linked to diseases such as Alzheimer's, various types of cancer, and heart disease. Aspirin is also a natural blood thinner, in fact, some cardiologists recommend that their patients take baby aspirin every other day. However, before you start popping aspirin indiscriminately, you should know that aspirin is not a benign substance. The same prostaglandins that cause inflammation everywhere else in the body have a protective effect on the lining of the stomach. Regular use of aspirin can cause gastrointestinal bleeding and ulcers and may be responsible for up to 33,000 deaths each year. Personally, I feel that aspirin must be used with caution. If you use aspirin everyday, take a baby aspirin.

If you take aspirin, beware of using other blood thinners, like vitamin E or ginkgo biloba. The combination could cause a bleeding problem.

Possible Benefits

Enhances the effect of ephedra.
Reduces inflammation.
May prevent heart disease, and reduce the risk of cancer.

How to Use It

A baby aspirin if you must take it daily. The usual dose for the ECA stack is much higher—three 300 mg. tablets daily. I warn you—proceed with caution!

Caution

Aspirin can deplete your levels of folic acid , vitamin C, and zinc. If you take aspirin regularly, be sure to take a multivitamin.

ASTAXANTHIN

There's a lot of buzz about this new antioxidant supplement, and there's some interesting science behind it that makes it stand out from the crowd. *Astaxanthin* is a member of the carotenoid family, natural pigments found in both plants and animals. Although there are seven hundred carotenoids in nature, there are only sixty present in food. Astaxanthin is produced by some algae and yeast, and provides the pink coloring to salmon, trout, and shrimp. Recent studies show that astaxanthin is a powerful antioxidant that may

reduce muscle soreness and speed recovery after a rigorous workout—
at least it did in preliminary studies. Considering what we know about
the role of antioxidants in exercise and muscle damage (see "Antioxidants"), this makes perfect sense. The question is, is this particular antioxidant appreciably better than others, like vitamin E? Studies of
animal cells suggest that astaxanthin is more effective against a particularly potent form of free radical (singlet oxygen) than vitamin E. Of
course, whether it works that way within the human body is still unknown. Several other studies performed by reputable scientists document that astaxanthin protects against lipid peroxidation in test tube
studies. *Lipid peroxidation*—the oxidation of fat in the body—is a major
cause of heart disease, but that's not all. Our brains contain high
amounts of fatty tissue: The oxidation of lipids in the brain could be a
major cause of brain aging. In my opinion, antioxidants that can protect
against the rusting of lipids in the body are worth their weight in gold.

Numerous studies have also found that astaxanthin is a natural immune booster that can protect animals against various types of cancer.
It is also an anti-inflammatory. Unlike many antioxidants, astaxanthin
can cross the blood–brain barrier, meaning that it is taken up by nerve
cells in the brain. Researchers have speculated that it may also be useful
to treat degenerative nerve diseases and macular degeneration of the
eye, as well as Parkinson's disease.

As interesting as astaxanthin may be, I'd like to see a few more
human studies before I wholeheartedly recommend it. By the way, I
don't recommend any carotenoid supplement, including this one, for
smokers. A major study showed that smokers who took beta carotene,
another carotenoid, were more likely to get cancer than those who
didn't. I have no idea whether astaxanthin would help or hurt smokers
but, since we don't know the answer, I suggest that smokers steer clear
of this one. (And, yes, do quit as soon as you can.)

One more thing. Whenever a new performance product is introduced to the public, manufacturers tend to go over the top, with ads
claiming that it's going to make you bigger and better. I don't know
what the manufacturers are going to say about this stuff, but I can tell
you that it may make you healthier, it may help save your heart and your
brain, and, yes, it may even reduce those post-workout aches and pains,

but there's no evidence that it will make you bigger. Sorry: If that's all you're interested in, save your money.

Possible Benefits

Protects against free radicals.
Speeds up post-workout recovery.

How to Use It

Take two 1 mg. tablets daily.

....

BEE POLLEN
....

 Pollen is gathered from the *stamen* (the male seed) of flowers by bees and stored in bee hives. Pollen is carried from flower to flower in a process called *pollination*. In fact, bees fertilize 80 percent of the plants on the planet! The leftover pollen remains in the hive and is deposited in honeycomb. If you're allergic, you've undoubtedly heard of pollen, and know that on days when the pollen count is high, you are likely to feel miserable. However, when ingested, bee pollen may actually be good for you. Since ancient times, bee pollen has been revered as the ultimate health food. According to Norse legends, it was the secret to eternal life and, in the Middle East, it was called the ambrosia of the gods. In fact, in 1972, Finnish runners attributed their unprecedented 5,000 meter and 10,000 meter gold medals at the Munich Olympic games to their regular use of bee pollen. Since then, bee pollen has been touted as a super-food and cure-all for nearly every ailment, ranging from fatigue to obesity to enlarged prostate. Recent studies suggest that some of these claims may be right on target!

Dubbed nature's most complete food, bee pollen contains an impressive array of nutrients, including twenty-two amino acids, bioflavonoids, natural antibiotics, enzymes, hormones, natural sugars called *glucosides*, vitamins, minerals, and essential fatty acids. It is especially rich in B vitamins (no pun intended). For more than two decades, Soviet athletes have extolled the virtues of bee pollen as the ultimate performance supplement. Soviet studies conducted in the 1970s and 1980s report that bee pollen enhances both stamina and performance, especially for endurance athletes. Only recently, however, have Western scientists taken a serious look at bee pollen, and they are finding a scientific basis for the claims.

Recent animal studies suggest that bee pollen may prove to be an effective weapon in the battle of the bulge. In a study conducted at Northeastern Ohio University College of Medicine and St. Thomas Hospital in Akron, Ohio, researchers fed laboratory rats either a diet consisting of bee pollen or laboratory chow over a twelve-week period. Both sets of rats were thriving on their diets. There was one major difference between the bee-pollen–fed animals and the chow-fed animals: The bee-pollen–fed animals had significantly less body fat and more lean tissue! Can bee pollen do the same for humans? Although there are no studies of bee pollen's effect on human metabolism, anecdotal reports suggest that it may help control appetite. Two tablespoons contain about ninety calories—that's a lot of nutrition packed into a small package. Those who take bee pollen claim that it boosts energy and stamina.

A standardized, patented form of bee pollen has been used successfully as a treatment for prostate enlargement and prostatitis. First used in Europe, bee pollen is now included in natural remedies for prostate problems in the United States. Bee pollen is also reputed to increase sperm count and enhance fertility in men.

Although many allergic people can tolerate oral bee pollen (it's just the stuff that floats around that gives them trouble), there have been reports of people developing severe allergic reactions to oral bee pollen. Therefore, I suggest that if you have any allergies at all, start with a small amount to see if it agrees with you. Begin with one-eighth teaspoon and, if you have no allergic reaction, gradually increase the amount you ingest until you reach your maximum dose.

Severely allergic people should not use bee pollen. Interestingly, some alternative physicians use bee pollen as a treatment for allergies, but I would not recommend this unless you are working with a skilled physician.

Possible Benefits

Energy booster.

May help control appetite and/or burn fat.

Natural remedy for prostate problems.

How to Use It

Bee pollen is sold in powder and capsules. Take one to three 500 mg. capsules daily. I recommend that you start with a low dose (one-half teaspoon sprinkled on cereal or fruit) to see if you have any allergic reaction. Gradually increase your dose to two table-spoons daily. Don't cook bee pollen—heat destroys many of its important nutrients.

BETA SITOSTEROL

 Beta sitosterol is one of the most misunderstood supplements on the market today. Some manufacturers claim that it is a potent anabolic substance that works as well as steroids. It's supposed to pump you up and send testosterone levels soaring. This is nonsense! There is absolutely no evidence that it builds muscle or boosts testosterone. When I contacted a manufacturer and asked them to produce some studies that can prove these claims, they never returned my calls and emails. As a result of these over-the-top claims, the experts who review supplements for body builders dismiss beta sitosterol as worthless. The fact is that it's not worthless. It does other things that are good for you, and you should know about them.

Beta sitosterol belongs to a family of phytochemicals called *phytosterols*, chemicals that are similar to cholesterol present in plants. For reasons that are not fully understood, beta sitosterol (and other phytosterols) can lower elevated cholesterol levels. In fact, sex claims for beta sitosterol may be related to its cholesterol-cutting activity. High cholesterol is an indicator of clogged arteries that could result in poor circulation, which can affect sexual performance. There are other ways that beta sitosterol may have been linked to improved sexual performance. Beta sitosterol is also a natural anti-inflammatory that reduces the level of *prostaglandins*, hormonelike substances that contribute to inflammation. Interestingly, beta sitosterol is found in *pygeum*, an herb well known for its treatment of enlarged prostate (BPH), a problem which is greatly aggravated by inflammation! Interestingly, pygeum is also reputed to be an aphrodisiac. Although BPH doesn't interfere with sexual performance *per se*, it can be an extremely uncomfortable problem that keeps you running to the bathroom constantly. That certainly can take the zip out of your sex drive!

Many herbs rich in plant sterols (such as sarsaparilla and avena sativa) are also touted as testosterone boosters and sex enhancers. Now you understand why!

More good news about beta sitosterol—animal studies show that it has some cancer-fighting properties. Beta sitosterol is indeed worthwhile, but don't expect miracles.

Possible Benefits

Lowers high cholesterol.
Good for prostate health.

How to Use It

Take one 30 mg. capsule daily. Beta sitosterol is also included in formulas for male health. Eat pumpkin seeds—they're a great source of beta sitosterol. I take a prostate formula that contains beta sitosterol.

BOSWELLIA

Are you sore after a workout? Do your joints ache from excessive wear and tear? This ancient Indian herb may help soothe those annoying trouble spots. *Boswellia serrata*, a tree that grows in the mountainous regions of India, is part of the ancient Ayurvedic system of medicine. Traditionally, it's been used as a treatment for a wide array of ailments, ranging from hemorrhoids to hair loss to heart disease, but it is best known as a treatment for inflammatory conditions and arthritis.

If you routinely take NSAIDs to relieve postexercise pain, I recommend that you try boswellia. When tested against NSAIDs, boswellia was shown to be as effective, but without any of the troublesome side effects, like gastric distress. In a study conducted by the Indian Council for Scientific and Industrial Research, 175 patients with rheumatoid arthritis were given either 450–750 mg. of boswellia daily or *Ketoprofen*, a commonly used NSAID. The patients taking the boswellia reported a significant decrease in joint pain and swelling, as did the patients taking the NSAID, but the boswellia patients did not have any of the unpleasant side effects experienced by NSAID users.

In another Indian study, boswellia was tested on patients with osteoarthritis, the most common form of this ailment. Here, too, boswellia passed with flying colors. Patients reported that it relieved pain, reduced morning stiffness, and improved grip strength.

Boswellia is often included in oral formulas for arthritis, as well as in creams that can be rubbed directly into painful areas. As with other herbs, it may take a bit longer for the pain-relieving properties of boswellia to kick in compared to NSAIDs but, in the long run, it may work as well for you without side effects.

Possible Benefits

Relieves sore muscles.
Reduces symptoms of arthritis.

How to Use It

Internal use: Take three 500 mg. capsules daily.
External use: Rub Boswellia cream on sore joints.

BRANCHED-CHAIN AMINO ACIDS

Amino acids are the building blocks of protein, essential for the production, maintenance, and repair of all living cells. Protein is required to make blood, antibodies, enzymes, muscle, and just about everything else within the body. The daily value for protein is 50 grams, but numerous studies confirm that endurance athletes and bodybuilders require more protein than sedentary folks. This makes sense—the more intense your workout, the more you beat up your muscles, and the more protein you need to repair them. There are twenty-two different amino acids. Fourteen can be made by the body, and are called *nonessential* or *dispensable* amino acids. Eight cannot be made by the body and, therefore, must be obtained through food or supplements. These are called *essential* or *indispensable* amino acids. (A ninth amino acid, *histidine*, is essential for infants and children, but not adults.)

Branched-chain amino acids (BCAAs) are three essential amino acids—leucine, isoleucine, and valine. Their unique chemical structure sets them apart from other amino acids, which makes them of particular importance to weight lifters and endurance athletes. Under normal circumstances, carbohydrates are burned as fuel but, during an intense workout, when you are placing unusual work demands on your body, protein may be broken down and burned as fuel. Due to their molecular structure, BCAAs are readily converted into glucose. In fact, during an intense workout, up to 10 percent of all energy comes from BCAAs. As every body builder knows, the more protein you burn for energy, the less protein there is available for muscle repair and to build new muscle. Therefore, you need enough BCAAs on hand to burn for energy without depleting your ability to synthesize more protein. Dairy products, red meat, whey protein, and eggs are rich in BCAAs but, during times of physical stress (like running a marathon) or intense exercise, you may need more than you can get from food alone.

Although researchers have not been able to link BCAA supplementation to improved performance, several studies have found supplemental BCAAs to be beneficial to people who frequently overtax their bodies. In one Swedish study, seven male endurance-trained cyclists were either given supplemental BCAAs in flavored water or a placebo during a period of intense exercise. During the times the cyclists were given BCAA-laced water, their ratings of perceived exhaustion were 7 percent lower, and their ratings of mental fatigue 15 percent lower than when they were given the placebo. Although BCAAs did not affect athletic endurance, they helped these athletes maintain their mental energy, which could prove important for sports in which mental focus is as critical as physical prowess.

In another Swedish study, researchers investigated whether supplemental BCAAs could prevent the breakdown of muscle. Researchers at the Karolinska Institute in Stockholm gave cross-country runners 7.5 grams BCAAs mixed in a 5 percent–carbohydrate drink in five doses throughout a 30-km. race. The researchers reported that the supplemental BCAAs raised the concentration of BCAAs in the blood as compared to a carbohydrate placebo, which suggests that more BCAAs could be burned as energy, sparing precious protein needed to build muscle.

If you're looking to trim down around the waist, take note. In an intriguing Italian study of competitive collegiate wrestlers on weight-loss diets, researchers reported that those taking BCAA supplementation lost more weight and, in particular, more body fat, than those not taking BCAAs. In particular, the BCAA supplemented group had a greater reduction in abdominal fat!

Possible Benefits

Helps spare protein needed to build and repair muscles.
Reduces mental fatigue associated with intense exercise.
May help burn fat, and reduce abdominal fat as part of a weight-loss diet and exercise regimen.

How to Use It

Replenish your supply of BCAAs one hour before to one hour after working out.
Take 2–4 grams daily. (Whey powder* is also an excellent source of BCAAs.)

CAFFEINE

There's no doubt that caffeine is the most popular recreational drug in the world. A cup of java, a strong cup of tea, or a cola drink gives you an instant lift. Caffeine is a central nervous system stimulant—it wakes you up and improves concentration and mental focus, at least temporarily. It boosts levels of stress hormones *epinephrine* and *norepinephrine*, which makes you alert, and blocks a chemical in the brain, which promotes sleep. Caffeine also increases the level of a brain hormone called *dopamine*, which makes you feel good.

Some people can tolerate caffeine better than others. For people who are caffeine sensitive, a cup or two of coffee will send their hearts racing and their heads pounding. So, as with anything else, if you use caffeine, you need to know your limits.

Caffeine has been used as a stimulant for thousands of years, but it is best known these days for its role in the ECA stack (ephedra, caffeine, aspirin) used for weight loss. Several studies have documented that 200 mg. caffeine taken with 20 mg. ephedrine three times daily one hour before meals can produce greater weight loss than ephedra used alone, or a placebo. (200 mg. of caffeine is equivalent to two six-ounce cups filtered, drip coffee or four six-ounce cups instant coffee, or eight six-ounce cups cola.)

For some people, caffeine can be addictive. If you're used to having several cups of coffee daily, a day without coffee can be a day with a splitting headache! So, when you go off your ECA stack, you may have similar withdrawal symptoms.

Personally, I don't use caffeine, I don't like the way it makes me feel. In most cases, however, two to three cups of coffee or tea daily isn't going to hurt you. In terms of enhancing performance, however, I think there are a lot of supplements better and safer than caffeine. I strongly advise against taking caffeine pills or using highly caffeinated products. For one thing, the energizing effect of caffeine is very short-lived—you'll crash within a few hours. Second, if you have a hidden heart problem, these products could kill you. So, steer clear.

Possible Benefits

Boosts metabolism.
Increases alertness.

How to Use It

If you must use caffeine, I recommend that you get your caffeine fix in the form of green tea.* It does everything caffeine should, but it also protects against cancer and heart disease. It comes in the multiple-antioxidant formula that I take twice daily with food.

CALCIUM

 If you're an endurance or strength athlete, you're constantly pushing your body to its limit. You work it hard to achieve optimal results. Because you expect so much from your body, you need to take care of it better than the average person. In particular, you need to make sure that you are getting enough nutrients. If you're like most athletes, however, you're not getting enough calcium. You could end up paying a steep price for this deficiency down the road.

Calcium does a lot of good things in your body, and it is absolutely essential for the formation of bone. During the first three decades of life, we are in bone-building mode. From our thirties on, we are constantly trying maintain the bone we have but, by our fifties, we begin to lose bone mass. If you lose too much bone, you run the risk of developing *osteoporosis*, characterized by the thinning of bone, making it vulnerable to breaks and shrinkage. (You can actually lose a few inches of height.) Obviously, it's critical to lay down enough bone when you're young so you have some to spare in your later decades, and that means getting enough calcium *now*. A recent study of ten thousand female athletes age seven to fifty revealed that less than half of them consumed 1000 mg. calcium daily. (Depending on your age, the recommended intake of calcium ranges from 1000–1500 mg. daily.) Teenage athletes of both sexes need to be concerned about getting enough calcium. Excessive training can lower levels of key hormones: Levels of estrogen dip in young female athletes, as do levels of testosterone in male athletes. Since these hormones are also critical for bone formation, the decline in hormones could lead to premature osteoporosis. This problem is compounded by the fact that so many young athletes are watching their weight to the point that they are following very low-calorie diets that don't provide enough nutrients. Many athletes have *bona fide* eating disorders. Obviously, it's important for coaches to avoid overtraining young athletes, but it's also essential for young athletes to be encouraged to eat well, get enough calcium rich foods, or take supplements.

Men and women over fifty also need to be vigilant about getting enough calcium. You need about 1200 mg. daily! I don't claim calcium alone can prevent osteoporosis, but it's certainly one of the important nutrients you need. Calcium is not just for strong bones; it is also important for normal cell function, and may protect against high blood pressure, heart disease, and colon cancer. New research also shows that calcium can help with weight control.

Possible Benefits

Helps build bone, may prevent or lessen the severity of osteoporosis.

How to Use It

Athletes require 1200 mg. calcium daily. Postmenopausal women not on hormone-replacement therapy should take 1500 mg. daily. (Look for calcium in the form of hydroxyapatite and purified glycinated calcite.)

CARNITINE

facts *Carnitine* is an amino-acidlike substance produced in the body and found in food. Lamb and beef have high amounts of carnitine; vegetables have very little. In the body, carnitine is synthesized from two essential amino acids, lysine and methionine, as well as vitamins C and B6, and iron. (L-carnitine is the preferred, natural form of carnitine.) If you are deficient in any of these building blocks of carnitine, you may not make enough carnitine. First used in Italy, carnitine created a buzz in 1982 when the Italian soccer team attributed its world-championship win to carnitine supplementation. Athletes began taking carnitine in the mistaken belief that it could make them instant, world-class winners. When it failed to live up to the hype, carnitine fell out of favor, at least for a while. New scientific research, however, has lent support to the use of carnitine as a tool for better sports performance. Like everything else, however, carnitine works best in conjunction with a training program, good nutrition, and other supplements.

Carnitine is essential for the production of energy within the body. Carnitine transports fatty acids into the mitochondria, the so-called powerhouse of the cell where energy is produced. Carnitine is often compared to the fuel pump in an automobile. Your body can have all the essential ingredients necessary to make energy but, without carnitine, they cannot get into the mitochondrial engines where the conversion into energy takes place. Carnitine is also essential for the production of muscle. First, without energy, the body cannot perform any task, including making new cells or repairing old ones. Second, carnitine provides the chemical backbone for the production of hormones, including anabolic hormones, like testosterone. Third, studies have shown that carnitine helps control the toxic effects of cortisol on brain cells and, although it hasn't been studied, it very likely has the same protective effect on muscle cells. (Long-term exposure to high levels of cortisol can break down lean tissue.)

Carnitine is also important for endurance sports. Intense exercise produces a significant drop in muscle carnitine levels; taking supplementary carnitine can help prevent that loss. Studies have shown that carnitine supplementation increases the maximum use of oxygen in athletes, allowing them to work out longer without fatigue. Runners who take 2 grams of carnitine per day can increase their peak running speed by as much as 6 percent. Carnitine can also help relieve post-workout soreness. An Italian researcher reported that carnitine can protect against delayed-onset muscle soreness (DOMS), which occurs twenty-four to forty-eight hours after an intense workout. Unlike other performance supplements, carnitine appears to work well for nontrained people. In one Italian study, nonathletes who took carnitine performed significantly better on a bicycle ergonmeter than those taking a placebo.

Carnitine is also great for your heart. For more than a decade, physicians in Italy, Sweden and Japan have given carnitine to patients suffering from angina (chest pain) and heart disease, often with other therapies. Carnitine can lower elevated levels of triglycerides, which increase the risk of having a heart attack, and raise levels of beneficial HDL, which moves excess cholesterol out of the body.

Possible Benefits

Increases energy and endurance.
Helps speed recovery after an intense workout.
May help prevent heart disease.

How to Take It

Take 500–3000 mg. daily, one hour before or one hour after eating, for best results. There are two kinds of carnitine, L-carnitine and D-carnitine. Some studies suggest that D-carnitine may be toxic, therefore, stick to products containing L-carnitine or acetyl-l-carnitine.

CAROTENOIDS

If your fitness regimen includes spending a lot of time outdoors, you must protect your skin against the sun's damaging UV rays. Skin is not just decoration or a container; it's the largest organ system in the body and one of the hardest working. Skin provides covering and protection for our internal organs, and is our first line of defense against bacteria, viruses, and other foreign and toxic substances. Skin is the only organ that is constantly exposed to the environment and, because of this, it pays a steep price in terms of wear and tear. The constant exposure to pollutants and sun will not only age your skin prematurely, but can have serious consequences, most notably skin cancers.

Whenever you are exposed to sunlight, be sure to wear sunscreen that protects against both UVA and UVB rays. I recommend a sunscreen with an SPF (sun protection factor) of at least fifteen. It's not enough to just protect your skin from the outside; recent studies suggest that the best approach may be one that protects from the outside in *and* the inside out! *Carotenoids* are antioxidant chemicals found in brightly colored fruits and vegetables, ranging from brilliant yellow, red, and orange to purple and dark green. *Mixed carotenoids* are a combination supplement including several different carotenoids found in nature (such as alpha carotene, beta carotene, lycopene, lutein, cryptoxanthin, and zeaxanthin). A recent study published in the *American Journal of Clinical Nutrition* showed that natural mixed carotenoids can help protect skin against sun damage. In the groundbreaking study, eleven men and eleven women took natural mixed carotenoids for twenty-four weeks. They took 30 mg. per day for the first eight weeks, 60 mg. for the second eight weeks, and 90 mg. for the final eight weeks. After the first eight weeks, the researchers measured the skin's sensitivity to UV light. As the dose of mixed carotenoids was increased, the participant's skin became more resistant to sunburn. In addition, blood tests showed a decrease in free radicals, proving that carotenoids are also powerful antioxidants. In another study, also published in the *American Journal of Clinical Nutrition*, researchers reported that the combination of vitamin E with mixed carotenoids provided even more powerful protection against the sun.

Some studies suggest that carotenoids, particularly lutein, can protect your vision! Remember, exposure to UV radiation also contributes to the formation of cataracts and, possibly, macular degeneration.

Possible Benefits

Helps prevent sun damage that can lead to premature aging of skin and cancer.

How to Use It

Take 60–90 mg. natural mixed carotenoids daily.

Caution:

Do not use synthetic mixed carotenoid supplements if you smoke! Some studies suggest that the mix of cigarette smoke and synthetic carotenoids may promote the formation of free radicals. Of course, the best source of carotenoids are fresh fruits and vegetables. Better yet, stop smoking.

CAYENNE

 Yup, the same stuff that gives food a kick is becoming a hot peak performance herb. You'll find cayenne or *capsaicin* (its active ingredient) in antioxidant formulas, ointments, and rubs for muscle pain, fat burners, and anticellulite supplements. Cayenne has been used for thousands of years in traditional medicine, primarily for respiratory infections, fevers, and digestive problems. Although cayenne is reputed to cause gastrointestinal distress, in reality, it stimulates the production of gastric juices that improves digestion. (Of course, people with ulcers should steer clear of cayenne, which could irritate their stomach lining.) It's also a mild stimulant that warms you up, but only temporarily. It increases peripheral circulation, but actually lowers core body temperature. That's why people eat hot foods in hot climates—you feel a flush of warmth, but the net effect is cooling.

Cayenne helps improve circulation, which is why it's used in cellulite formulas, often along with natural diuretics and/or fat blockers or fat burners. Cellulite, those dimples on hips, thighs, and buttocks, is caused by a number of factors including genetics, hormones, and poor circulation. Although cayenne may help improve circulation, I don't think it's a cure for this problem. As far as its fat-burning potential is concerned, I think cayenne may be helpful along with other thermogenic supplements, but that the effect is relatively weak. I have not seen any studies to convince me otherwise.

Cayenne's main reason for being in your gym bag could be its ability to control pain. Capsaicin blocks the production of *substance P*, which triggers pain and inflammation. Capsaicin creams have been used successfully to treat arthritis, diabetic neuropathy, and cluster headaches. If you have a tennis elbow or jogger's knee that's giving you problems, especially after you work out, try rubbing capsaicin cream over the affected area.

Possible Benefits

Increases metabolism.
Improves digestion.
Soothes painful joints.

How to Use It

Internal use: Take up to three capsules daily to improve circulation and digestion.

External use: Rub ointment directly on sore joints and muscles.

CHONDROITIN

 Chondroitin sulfate is the lesser known half of the dynamic supplement duo known as the *arthritis cure* (glucosamine plus chondroitin sulfate.) Although it's played second fiddle to the better known glucosamine, chondroitin sulfate is in a class by itself. Chondroitin sulfate is a major constituent of *cartilage*, the thin, smooth substance that lines the joints and prevents bones from rubbing against each other. Age and overuse can wear down cartilage, resulting in osteoarthritis, also known as wear-and-tear arthritis. Although osteoarthritis tends to strike people in their later years, if you continually beat up your joints (if you lift heavy weights, or jog on hard pavement, or live on the Stairmaster), you may get osteoarthritis in vulnerable joints even earlier.

Osteoarthritis can be very painful. Millions of people turn to nonsteroidal anti-inflammatory medications (NSAIDs) to relieve the pain, although these drugs often cause serious gastrointestinal problems, including bleeding and ulcers. Several studies in leading medical journals confirm that chondroitin sulfate is very effective in relieving the aches and pains associated with arthritis, with virtually no side effects. A study in the *Journal of Rheumatology* (January 2000) tested chondroitin sulfate against a placebo on osteoarthritis patients. Patients who took the placebo reported a 20 percent improvement (which shows the power of a placebo), but patients who took chondroitin showed a 60 percent reduction in pain within a three to six month period, which shows the power of chondroitin. Chondroitin attracts fluid to cartilage, providing shock absorption for the surrounding bones and bathing the joint in healing nutrients.

There is another good reason to take chondroitin. Chondroitin is present in the lining of blood vessels, and may lower high blood-cholesterol levels. In animal studies, chondroitin helped to prevent atherosclerosis, the clogging of the arteries by plaque that can lead to a heart attack.

Animal studies suggest that chondroitin can help repair broken bones, but there have not been similar studies in humans. Nevertheless, if you have a broken bone, there's no reason not to take chondroitin—it may help mend you faster.

Unless you eat a lot of meat gristle, you don't get much chondroitin from food. Fortunately, your body makes chondroitin but, if you've got osteoarthritis, you need chondroitin supplements.

Chondroitin appears to work in synergy with glucosamine. When combined, these two peak performance supplements can reduce pain of osteoarthritis, and may even stimulate the regeneration of cartilage. For best results, take the arthritis helper at the first sign of osteoarthritis.

Possible Benefits

Relieves symptoms of osteoarthritis.
May protect against heart disease.

How to Use It

Take up to two 500 mg. capsules daily.

CHROMIUM

Chromium is a trace mineral found in foods such as brewers yeast, lobster, liver, and black pepper. Chromium is important because it is part of the glucose tolerance factor, GTF, which helps regulates insulin and is involved in protein synthesis and helps control appetite. Chromium is also essential for proper glucose and lipid metabolism. The more sugar you consume, the more chromium your body needs. I'm not just talking about the few spoonfuls of sugar you put in your coffee, or the occasional chocolate bar you may eat. Sugar is a staple of our modern, processed food supply. It's in soda, bread, cakes, cookies, and in places where you would least expect it, like pasta sauce, so-called health cereals, and canned fruit and soups. Unfortunately, it's very difficult to get enough chromium from food alone. Chances are, you do not get the 50 mcg. chromium established as the minimal safe and adequate intake by the National Academy of Sciences (about 90 percent of Americans don't).

If you engage in vigorous exercise, you may also need more chromium. Chromium helps the body use insulin more efficiently, which is essential for the preservation and creation of skeletal muscle. Insulin directs amino acids into muscle cells, where they are made into proteins needed to repair and produce more muscle cells. Insulin also slows the breakdown of protein *(catabolism)* leaving more protein available for building muscle. Baby boomers, beware! Due to our unhealthy diet and sedentary lifestyle, insulin resistance is a virtual epidemic in the United States, and you are at risk. Also called *Type II diabetes*, in the case of insulin resistance, there is plenty of insulin, but the hormone works less efficiently. At least 25 percent of all U.S. adults develop some form of insulin resistance and, not surprisingly, most are overweight and flabby. The risk of developing insulin resistance rises exponentially with each passing decade after age thirty. By age seventy you are twenty times more likely to develop Type II diabetes than you were at age fifty. As the risk of insulin resistance rises, studies show that blood levels of chromium decline as well. In fact, some researchers believe that the drop in chromium is responsible for the rise in insulin resistance. For nearly two decades, researchers have been studying chromium as a treatment for insulin resistance, and it was this work that led to an increased understanding of chromium's role in helping to maintain a trim, fit body.

Chromium supplementation works best for two groups of people—the moderately obese and the superfit. In one study of 154 moderately obese people (25 percent over ideal body weight), those who took 200–400 mcg. chromium daily for seventy-two days without changing their diet or exercising patterns lost an average of 4.2 pounds of fat, compared to just .04 pounds of fat lost in the placebo group. However, when chromium was given to normal weight healthy people, it did not result in a loss of fat or a gain in muscle.

In another study, researchers gave young athletes 400 mcg. chromium. At the end of twenty-four weeks of rigorous aerobic training, the athletes showed a 3.5 percent increase in lean body mass and a decrease in body fat of 4.6 percent, as compared to those taking a placebo. A similar study in which football players were given 200 mcg. chromium over eight weeks did not show any improvement in body composition. For the very fit, chromium works best at the higher dose, and takes longer to produce results.

Chromium is one of the few supplements that can raise the level of HDL, or good cholesterol, which helps protect against heart disease. It has also been used quite successfully to treat Type II diabetes in China as part of a study sponsored by the U.S. Department of Agriculture.

The effects of chromium are subtle and long term. It is not going to bulk you up overnight, or make you slim. If you are overweight, it will help tone up your physique (especially if you exercise and watch what you eat). If you are engaged in a rigorous training program, chromium is another tool that will help preserve muscle.

Possible Benefits

Helps insulin work more efficiently.
Helps maintain muscle and burn fat.
May prevent insulin resistance.
Good for your heart!

How to Use It

Take 200–600 mcg. dinicotinate glycinate form of chromium daily.

CHRYSIN

Chrysin (Flavone X) is a phytochemical found in passion-flower, an herb I consider to be one of nature's best tranquilizers. Ironically, you're not supposed to take chrysin to wind down, it's supposed to help you bulk up! However, there's a lot of controversy as to whether it works at all. Chrysin is an isoflavone, an estrogenlike compound found in plants, including soy foods, lentils, and whole grains. Why would a guy want to take something that remotely resembles estrogen? For the same reason that women take isoflavones—to control the estrogen naturally produced in their bodies. In women, isoflavones are believed to inhibit the effect of potent estrogens that can stimulate the growth of estrogen sensitive tumors, like breast cancers. These compounds may also offer some of the positive benefits of estrogen without the side effects. What you may not know is that men also make estrogen. You need some estrogen to survive; your brain can't work without it. In men, testosterone is converted into estrogen through the action of an enzyme called *aromatase*. The key is to maintain the right balance between estrogen and testosterone. As men age, they make more estrogen and less testosterone, which can make them less muscular, tired, flabbier, less interested in sex, and generally depressed. At any age, if you are taking supplements to boost testosterone, you also run the risk of making more estrogen. In fact, a recent study suggest that andro elevates levels of estradiol, a potent estrogen. The buzz is that chrysin may block the action of aromatase, leaving you more free testosterone. At least, it appeared to work in test tube studies involving human cells, but that's a far cry from working inside the human body. Due to lack of scientific research, I can't say whether it works. One problem is that chrysin may not be easily absorbed by the body, and much of it may be excreted before it can do any good. Nevertheless, chrysin is included in many formulas containing testosterone-boosting supplements like andro and DHEA.

Chrysin is an antioxidant, and also has anti-inflammatory properties. Theoretically, it should help speed recovery of muscles after a workout.

Possible Benefits

May prevent the conversion of testosterone into estrogen.
If it works, could protect against hormone-sensitive cancers.

How to Use It

Take 1000–3000 mg. daily.

CIWUJIA

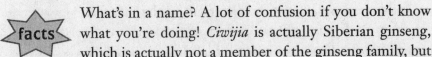

facts What's in a name? A lot of confusion if you don't know what you're doing! *Ciwijia* is actually Siberian ginseng, which is actually not a member of the ginseng family, but a related plant with many of the same properties. It is now being sold under its Chinese name, *ciwujia*. (Perhaps to make it sound more exotic?) Trust me, it's the same stuff. Not that there's anything wrong with Siberian ginseng. Russian studies confirm that this herb is a good ergonomic aid, and that it can increase strength and endurance. In fact, it's a favorite among Russian athletes. I've been writing about this herb for close to twenty years! Siberian ginseng is a tonic herb, which means it helps the body adjust to stressors of all kind—physical and emotional. Ciwujia is the primary ingredient in a popular sports supplement called Endurox, a standardized form of Siberian ginseng, but specially processed so that the stimulants are removed. Also produced by the same manufacturer, Endurance Excel combines 1200 mg. ciwujia with 60 IU vitamin E. The daily dose is two capsules. According to the manufacturer's studies, Endurox can increase fat metabolism by 43 percent, speed recovery from exercise, and build endurance. The presence of vitamin E in Endurance Excel is purported to speed recovery. Based on everything we know about ciwujia and vitamin E, these are reasonable claims. If you're looking for a mild energy boost, I think that ciwujia should help.

Unlike Asian ginseng, ciwujia doesn't cause insomnia—in fact, it's been used as a treatment for sleep problems. It won't make you jittery like real ginseng. In fact, ciwujia is a wonderful stress reliever. It's also an immune booster, and has been used for centuries to treat bronchitis and respiratory problems. If you are prone to colds and flus after a difficult training period, this supplement may help to keep you healthy.

Possible Benefits

Increases stamina.
Accelerates fat burning.
Speeds recovery from vigorous exercise.

How to Use It

Take two to three 400 mg. capsules daily. If you use a product containing ciwujia, follow the directions on the package.

CLA

In the 1970s, we counted calories and went to bed hungry. In the 1980s, we filled up on carbs and threw out the fat. In the 1990s, we piled our plates high with protein and threw out the carbs. You know what? None of it's worked! As a nation, we're getting fatter, flabbier, and sicker. It's no longer just a matter of middle-age spread; there's an alarming rise in obesity among all sectors of society, including elementary-school kids! Counting calories and fat grams, or slavishly following the diet *du jour*, has failed us. Clearly, we need a new approach to weight control and CLA may be just what the doctor ordered.

Conjugated linoleic acid is a fatty acid found in red meat and dairy products, or at least it used to be. . . . Grass grazed animals were rich in CLA but, due to modern farming practices, our food supply is now stripped of this fat. In fact, experts estimate that there has been an 80 percent decrease in CLA consumption since the 1960s, just about the time the nation's waistline began to collectively expand. Is there a connection? Some scientists believe that the loss of CLA in the diet could be directly related to the increase in obesity. Recent studies show that CLA can help burn fat and increase lean muscle tissue. Although manufacturers would have you believe that CLA is a magic pill that melts fat away practically overnight, it's not a fat cure. CLA may be a useful tool in helping people maintain a trim, sleek body, along with proper diet and exercise. It will not help you lose weight, but what it may do is help improve your muscle-to-fat ratio, which will make you look trimmer. Although animal studies have shown major changes in body composition in animals fed CLA, human studies have shown less dramatic changes. Nevertheless, there is compelling evidence that CLA may help maintain muscle mass. In one study conducted at Kent State University, researchers gave novice male body builders 7.2 grams daily of

CLA or a placebo. After six weeks of a body-building regimen, those who took the CLA showed more muscle and less fat in their arms than placebo takers. The researcher concluded that CLA was a mild anabolic agent. In another study conducted at the University of Memphis, researchers gave twenty-seven experienced resistance-trained males 5.6 grams CLA daily or a placebo. Although the researchers did not find that CLA altered body composition in these already-fit men, they did find something interesting. Supplementation reduced changes in the ratio of blood urea nitrogen to creatine, which indicates a catabolic or wasting state. In other words, this is an indication that CLA helps preserve muscle.

The benefits of CLA may extend far beyond the cosmetic. CLA may be a potent cancer fighter, as reported in a study published in *Anticancer Research*. In the study, mice were first fed a diet with 1 percent CLA or *linoleic acid*, a different type of fatty acid, for two weeks. Linoleic acid happens to be abundant in the western diet. The mice were then injected with a potent strain of human prostate cancer cells. After fourteen weeks, the mice were sacrificed. As expected, both groups of mice showed signs of tumor growth, but the CLA mice had significantly smaller tumors compared to the mice eating a linoleic-laced diet, or to mice in an earlier experiment that had not been given any additional fatty acids. Even more importantly, tumors in the mice fed CLA rarely spread to the lungs, whereas lung metastasis occurred in all the mice fed linoleic acid, and in 80 percent of mice not given any fatty acids. Other animal studies have shown that CLA can inhibit the growth of breast-cancer cells and, similar to the previous study, helped prevent the metastasis of breast cancer to the lungs and bone marrow. If CLA works as well in humans, it could be a useful preventive therapy against prostate and breast cancer.

Like omega-3 fatty acids, CLA can lower cholesterol and triglyceride levels, and improve insulin sensitivity, which can help reduce the risk of heart disease and diabetes.

Possible Benefits

Burns fat while sparing lean-muscle tissue.
May have anticarcinogenic activity.
Good for your heart.

How to Use It

Take up to three 1200 mg. capsules before meals.

. . . .

COLOSTRUM

. . . .

facts Can one little pill enhance stamina, boost immune function, burn fat, cure allergies, and build muscle? That's the promise of colostrum, a supplement that is supposed to do everything for everybody. Before you reject these claims as a lot of hype, there is some interesting science behind colostrum. Although it may not be the fountain of youth, as promoters claim, it is still worthy of the hot hundred.

Colostrum is *premilk*, a thin, yellowish fluid produced by lactating humans and mammals for only two days after giving birth. Commercial colostrum is derived from cow's milk (thus, it's sometimes called *bovine colostrum*). Endurance athletes take note: Colostrum is an excellent immune booster. Overtraining for a big race, or a particularly grueling workout, will deplete your immune function, at least temporarily, making you more vulnerable to colds and flus. Colostrum may be just the shot in the arm you need to stay well. It's well-known that mothers pass special immune protection onto their infants *via* breast milk. Colostrum contains the same immune-boosting substances, including *lactoferrin*, a natural antibiotic; and *immunoglobulins*, proteins that glob onto foreign invaders, targeting them for attack by other immune cells. In other words, if you take colostrum, you have a better shot at staying healthier. Colostrum is especially good at combating stomach bugs and so-called traveler's diarrhea.

There are conflicting studies as to whether colostrum can enhance athletic performance and build muscle. Colostrum's claim to fame is that it contains *growth factors*, substances that stimulate cell growth, repair, and healing. It raises levels of IGF, a hormone that mediates the activity of growth hormone, and, supposedly, can build muscle on its own. A recent study showed, however, that among weight lifters, IGF did not build muscle. However, a study of the Finnish Olympic ski team showed that when skiers took colostrum, it not only raised their levels of IGF, but resulted in faster muscle recovery after strenuous exercise. This suggests that something in colostrum has a mild muscle-sparing effect; whether its due to IGF is a subject of debate. IGF is also supposed to boost mood and, if not increase energy directly, at least produce an enhanced feeling of well-being.

If you routinely use nonsteroidal anti-inflammatory drugs (NSAIDs) for post-workout muscle pain or arthritis, you need to take colostrum. NSAIDs can damage the stomach lining, causing bleeding and ulcers. A recent study conducted at Leicester General Hospital in Leicester, England found that colostrum can protect the stomach lining against NSAID-induced damage.

Although, at this point, it's difficult to say whether colostrum is a true ergonomic aid. I am confident that colostrum can give your immune system more muscle. By the way, some people use colostrum face cream to prevent wrinkles and rejuvenate skin. It makes sense that the same growth factors that heal the stomach lining could improve the quality of skin.

Possible Benefits

Boosts immune function.
May accelerate muscle recovery.
May enhance wound healing.

How to Take It

Take three 480 mg. capsules daily on an empty stomach. When you are sick, you can take up to nine capsules daily.

CO-Q10

facts Co-Q10 (short for co-enzyme-Q10) is produced by every cell in the body. It is essential for energy production. Often called the biochemical sparkplug of the cell, Co-Q10 is found in the *mitochondria*, the powerhouse of the cell, where ATP is produced. ATP is the fuel that runs every bodily function, from thinking to running to the beating of your heart. When you work out hard, you go through a lot of ATP! Co-Q10 is also an antioxidant, important because one of the byproducts of energy production is free radicals, those overactive molecules that can attack and destroy healthy cells. The build up of free radicals in muscle can hamper recovery after a workout, and may cause long-term damage to muscles and joints. In fact, free radicals have been implicated as a risk factor in nearly every known disease, from heart attacks to Alzheimer's to arthritis. Having ample amounts of Co-Q10 and other antioxidants on hand may help prevent free radicals from running amuck.

Will taking Co-Q10 give you an energy boost? One study of twenty healthy male athletes showed it could improve exercise endurance over an eight-week period. This isn't to say, however, that taking Co-Q10 is going to produce a palpable energy surge. Co-Q10 will help keep a healthy body humming along, but it's not a pep pill! However, Co-Q10 offers so many other significant health benefits that I think it's important to include it in your daily supplement regimen.

One group of people who have shown dramatic improvement in energy levels after taking Co-Q10 are patients suffering from heart failure. The heart, which is arguably the hardest working organ of the body, is rich in energy-producing mitochondria. In the case of heart failure, the mitochondria become damaged, and do not produce adequate amounts of energy to keep the heart running well. Several studies have shown that Co-Q10 can help repair a sick heart and, in some cases, even reverse heart failure. These successful reports about Co-Q10's positive effect have led many people to believe (myself included) that taking Co-Q10 when you're healthy could be insurance against heart disease down the road.

Co-Q10 may prove to be the ultimate weapon against aging. A growing number of scientists believe that the aging process is actually a result of the slowdown in energy production by the cells. In fact, as mitochondria age, they begin to show signs of wear and tear, just like the rest of your body. Some scientists believe that taking Co-Q10 (often in combination with another peak performance supplement, carnitine) may tweak energy production, helping to prevent the telltale, age-related slowdown.

Co-Q10 is present in many different foods, but in particularly large quantities in organ meats, which are high in saturated fat; therefore, I don't recommend them. So, unless you're prepared to eat fourteen pounds of peanuts or six pounds of sardines a day to get my recommended dose, you'd better take supplements!

Possible Benefits

Helps to maintain energy production.
Good for your heart.
May slow down aging process.

How to Use It

Take one to three 30 mg. capsules daily with meals.

CORDYCEPS

facts *Cordyceps* (short for *Cordyceps sinensis*) is a rare Chinese mushroom that grows naturally on certain species of caterpillars. Fortunately, the cordyceps that are used today are cultivated through fermentation—that means, without caterpillars! For thousands of years, cordyceps have been used by Chinese healers as tonic for sexual vigor and overall vitality. It makes sense that cordyceps would be an effective aphrodisiac. Similar to ginkgo and other sex-enhancing herbs, cordyceps increases arterial blood flow, which sends more blood flowing to the pelvic area. According to Chinese studies, cordyceps can also improve athletic performance. A recent double-blind crossover study performed at St. Cloud State University in Minnesota confirms that, when combined with other tonic herbs, including Asian ginseng, enoki mushroom, green tangerine peel, reishi mushroom, and Siberian ginseng, cordyceps can speed recovery in athletes. (The specific formulation is sold under the name Metaflex and 2nd Wind.) In the study, twelve well-trained college athletes were either given a placebo or 950 mg. of the combination herbal formula for five weeks. At the end of the five weeks, the athletes cycled intensely for twenty minutes, rested for twelve minutes, then completed cycling. There was little difference in performance between the two groups, although those who took the herbs finished slightly faster than the placebo group. The real difference, however, was in the accumulation of lactic acid postexercise. Those who took the herbs had significantly less lactic-acid build up. As many of you know, *lactic acid* is a byproduct of glucose that builds up in muscles during anaerobic exercise (high-intensity exercise like weight-lifting or sprinting). Lactic acid buildup is what makes muscles sore after a hard workout. From this study, it's reasonable to assume that cordyceps may help speed recovery after intense exercise. Given its long-standing reputation as a tonic herb, it may also help relieve fatigue.

Possible Benefits

Reduces lactic acid buildup in muscles.
May enhance energy and stamina.

How to Use It

Take two 525 mg. capsules daily.

CREATINE

Of all the peak performance supplements, creatine is one of the most versatile and interesting. You've heard of creatine as the supplement that increases muscle mass and strength. Millions of serious athletes, like Sammy Sosa and Mark Mc-Gwire; school-aged athletes; and even weekend athletes are already using it. The Los Angeles Lakers are reputed to keep tubs of creatine in their locker room! What you may not know is that creatine also cuts high cholesterol and triglycerides, slows down tumor growth, and has even been used to prevent muscle wasting in AIDS patients.

Creatine is an amino acid found in meat and fish. Most people consume an average of 1 gram of creatine daily from food. Those who take creatine supplements take up to five grams a day—the equivalent of eating five to twenty-five pounds of meat daily!

First things first: You want to know if creatine can really transform a scrawny body into a powerhouse of strength? There have been more than three hundred studies on creatine since it was first brought to market in 1993. Most have been positive, with one caveat. Creatine works best when combined with rigorous exercise: It will enhance the effects of a workout, but it is not a magic muscle maker. For those who do work out, creatine seems to produce good results. The majority of studies have found that creatine can make muscles bigger and stronger, resulting in average weight gain of from two to three pounds. Typically, creatine produced a 5 to 10 percent increase in performance in activities involving sudden bursts of activity like sprinting. Remarkably, according to some studies, results can be seen within as little as five days. Most experts agree that creatine works by plumping up muscle cells with water (which makes them look bigger,) as well as helping to maintain lean muscle. Creatine is converted into creatine phosphate in the body, which is needed to recycle ADP to ATP (the body's fuel). Thus, it provides more ATP to muscle cells, enabling them to do more work. The highest concentrations of creatine are found in *fast-twitch muscle fibers*, the kind used to handle short-term, heavy-duty workloads, like sprinting and weight lifting.

In recent years, creatine has gotten some bad press, although much of it is undeserved. In 1997, creatine was reputed to have been involved in the deaths of three high-school wrestlers. The accusation was unfounded. A major newspaper later reported that the FDA had issued a warning about the use of creatine—that wasn't true either.

The biggest criticism about creatine is that it is so new that there are no long-term studies involving creatine users. In reality, creatine has been used to treat medical conditions for several decades. In fact, it was a 1981 article in the *New England Journal of Medicine* that reported the effect of creatine supplementation on patients with a rare visual problem that inadvertently triggered the creatine craze. The researcher noted that, although the patients taking creatine didn't show any improvement in the progression of their disease, it did produce a 10 percent increase in body weight, bigger muscles, and improved physical strength. (I wonder how many doctors started taking creatine after that report!) These patients have been followed for close to two decades, and have shown no adverse side effects. Yes, they still have better muscles. . . . Granted, this is not a large, double-blind study involving thousands of patients, but we do have the benefit of a real life clinical trial. Hundreds of thousands of people have been taking creatine for more than five years, and there are still no reports of any problems. My hunch is that creatine will prove to be safe for long-term use.

There have been sporadic reports of some minor, negative side effects, such as stomach upset, cramping, and an increased tendency toward muscle pulls, but these complaints have not shown up in most studies. I do not recommend creatine for people with kidney problems, since high amounts of protein can further stress the kidneys.

Creatine is not for every athlete. It's not particularly useful for endurance sports like marathon running. (You don't need the extra baggage!) It's best for high-intensity, short-duration exercise such as sprinting, football, weight lifting, and basketball, and is useful if you work out regularly (three times per week). I don't think that creatine does much for a weekend athlete.

There is some controversy as to whether high-school athletes should be allowed to use creatine—some coaches forbid it, others hand it out. Frankly, I think it's a lot safer than the other options, particularly hormone precursors like andro or speedlike ephedrine compounds.

Creatine monohydrate is the form of creatine that is most commonly used in supplements, because it is well absorbed by the body.

Possible Benefits

Helps build muscle.
Enhances physical performance for fast-action, high-intensity activities.
Reduces high cholesterol.

How to Use It

Creatine is sold in capsules, as a liquid, and in a powder, which can be mixed in water or juice. Start with a loading dose of 20–25 grams per day for five days. (Take 5–6 grams creatine up to four times daily with a meal or snack.) After five days, take 2 grams daily (one at breakfast and one at lunch). Creatine works best when combined with carbohydrate. Some studies suggest that caffeine can interfere with its effectiveness.

DHA

In Japan, students pop a DHA capsule or drink a DHA-laced beverage before taking exams. In the United States, some nutrition-minded pediatricians want it added to infant formula to make babies smarter! *Docosahexanenoic acid* (DHA) is a polyunsaturated omega-3 fatty acid that cannot be manufactured by the body, and must be obtained through foods such as fatty fish (tuna, salmon, and mackerel), organ meats, and eggs. DHA is found in high concentration in the gray matter of the brain and the retina of the eye. The cells of the brain communicate with each other by releasing chemicals called *neurotransmitters*, which is how thoughts and memories are transmitted. DHA helps keep brain-cell membranes fluid (permeable), which keeps the brain healthy and improves communication. Studies have shown that low blood levels of DHA have been linked to Alzheimer's disease, aggression, depression, and attention deficit hyperactivity disorder (ADHD). In fact, some studies have shown that DHA supplementation can enhance mental performance in healthy people as well as in people with severe dementia.

DHA is also present in breast milk, but not in most infant formula sold in the United States. You may have heard about studies that showed that children who had been breast fed have higher IQs than those who were not—many researchers believe this is due to a healthy dose of DHA in the crucial early years of brain development.

DHA is also believed to play an important role in mood. Studies have suggested that a low intake of DHA increases the risk of depression. In fact, in countries where fatty fish is eaten regularly, there is a much lower incidence of depression than in countries like the United States, where fatty fish is eaten less.

Possible Benefits

May give your brain a boost.
May give your mood a boost.

How to Use It

Take up to three 250 mg. capsules daily.

• •

DHEA

• •

facts Can dehydroepiandrosterone (DHEA) rev up your sex life? Recent studies suggest that this so-called superhormone can help you have a *super* sex life. DHEA is a steroid hormone found in abundance in the human body. DHEA is produced by the adrenal glands (located on the kidneys), as well as the brain and the skin. In fact, it is the most abundant steroid in the human body. As with estrogen and testosterone, levels of DHEA decline with age. DHEA levels rise steadily from puberty, peak at around age twenty, and then drop at about 2 percent per year. Many physicians and researchers believe that the drop in DHEA is in part responsible for the physical decline that we have long associated with aging, including weight gain, flabby muscles, loss of libido, and memory problems.

In a recent study published in the *New England Journal of Medicine*, twenty-four women with low adrenal function were given 50 mg. of DHEA daily for four months. After a month wash-out period (free of DHEA), the women were given a placebo for another four months. During the time the women were on DHEA, they reported feeling less depressed and anxious. They also noted a sharp increase in sex drive. DHEA seems to have the same effect on men. In another study, twenty men were given 50 mg. of DHEA for six months, another group of men was given a placebo. The men reported that DHEA not only increased their interest in sex, but noted an improvement in erectile dysfunction, orgasm, and overall satisfaction.

Although these studies did not find any untoward side effects of DHEA, there is one potential problem: DHEA breaks down in the body into two other hormones, estrogen and testosterone. It's possible that women could end up with too much testosterone, and men with too much estrogen. That's why men often take DHEA with other supplements (like chrysin, ipriflavone, and DIM), that are reputed to block the conversion of testosterone to estrogen. Women who take DHEA often take it in combination with estrogen to counterbalance testosterone. Physicians who prescribe DHEA say that, if given in the right doses, DHEA should not upset the normal hormonal balance. There is only one way you can be sure that you are taking the right dose of DHEA. You must have your hormone levels checked periodically by your doctor. This is the safest and best way to use DHEA.

DHEA also appears to control *cortisol*, the stress hormone that, if produced in excess, can sap you of your energy and make you depressed. High cortisol levels can also make your body retain fat, especially around the middle. As women age, they seem to gain weight around the waist. By controlling cortisol, DHEA may help prevent this unwanted weight gain.

Possible Benefits

Enhances sex drive in men and women.
Improves mood.

How to Use It

The usual dose is 25 mg. daily for women and 50 mg. daily for men. If you are over fifty, have your DHEA levels checked by a nutritional-oriented practitioner.

DHT BLOCKERS

 If you take a supplement that boosts testosterone levels—or if you take real testosterone—you could also be inadvertently boosting levels of a very potent form of testosterone, dihydrotestosterone. *Dihydrotestosterone* (DHT) is the hormone that enlarges the prostate gland (the walnut-shaped gland that surrounds the part of the urethra located under the bladder). It can also stimulate the growth of prostate cancer. To add insult to injury, it can even make you bald! Obviously, it's critical to control your levels of DHT. Guys over forty take note: Levels of DHT rise with age, which is why so many older men have prostate problems. You have to be extra careful about taking supplements or drugs that are going to send your DHT levels soaring. At the same time, you want to boost your levels of real testosterone so that you can increase strength, grow muscle, and maintain your libido. It's a delicate balance, and DHT blockers may help prevent the damaging effect of the dark side of testosterone.

There are several natural DHT blockers, including two well-known herbs: saw palmetto and pygeum. These herbs appear to work by inhibiting an enzyme that converts testosterone to DHT—5-alpha-reductase. They have been used successfully in men with BPH (benign prostate hypertrophy) and, frankly, given the current prostate cancer epidemic in the United States, I think all men should use them. Supplement manufacturers market them to athletes as the antidote to excess DHT and, although they never say it outright, suggest that they can also block the negative effects of anabolic steroids. Frankly, I seriously doubt it. Herbs are gentle medicine. Saw palmetto and pygeum work well for men with normal prostate problems who have normally elevated levels of DHT, but there are no studies that prove that they are any match for chemically induced DHT highs. When you mess around with strong drugs, prescription or otherwise, there are consequences. My advice is: Proceed with caution.

By the way, pygeum is reputed to be an aphrodisiac. One study said that men who took it reported an improvement in their ability to achieve an erection.

Possible Benefits

May help control DHT.

How to Use It

The usual dose is up to three 500 mg. capsules daily of each herb.

DIM

Diidolylmethane (DIM) is one of the newest and hottest peak performance supplements today, and you'll never guess where it comes from. It is a phytochemical found in cruciferous vegetables such as broccoli, cauliflower, cabbage, and brussels sprouts. DIM is formed from another important phytochemical, indole-3-carbinol, which gained fame a decade ago as a possible cancer fighter. Indole-3-carbinol was shown to inactivate potent estrogens that promote the growth of tumors in estrogen-sensitive cells (like breast cells.) Indole-3-carbinol increases the body's production of 2-hydroxy estrogen and 2-hydroxy estrone, good estrogens that are antioxidants and may protect against cancer. It also blocks the production of bad estrogens. However, indole-3-carbinol can't do its good work without first being converted to DIM, which occurs in the digestive tract. So why not just eat your veggies? You'd have to eat about one and a half pounds of broccoli daily to get a significant hormone-balancing benefit! Fortunately, Michael Zeligs, M.D., of Boulder, Colorado has developed a form of DIM that can be taken as a tablet.

Clearly this is big news for women, but why should guys care about estrogen? Men make estrogen, too (it's produced in the adrenal glands from testosterone) although in smaller quantities than do women. High levels of potent estrogens can cause serious problems for men, and have been associated with an increased risk of prostate cancer. Men who take testosterone, DHEA, or T-boosters may inadvertently also be boosting their levels of these potent estrogens. They are not only increasing their risk of cancer, but may develop some nasty side effects like fuller breasts. Manufacturers of DIM products for men contend that it increases the activity of free testosterone, which means there is more testosterone available for energy and muscle building.

For more about DIM, I recommend that you read Dr. Zeligs's book, *All About DIM*.

Possible Benefits

Protects against potent estrogen.
May increase free testosterone.

How to Use It

Take up to two 200 mg. tablets daily.

NATURAL DIURETICS

facts Diuretics are substances that help the body shed excess water weight. Natural diuretics derived from herbs have become popular as weight-loss tools. They are used by body builders who are trying to lose every drop of water for that sleek, defined look, and by women with PMS who can't fit into their clothes because of bloating, and by dieters looking for any way to tip the scale in their favor. Natural diuretics include dandelion, uva ursi, buchu, and celery seed. They are sold alone or in combination formulas. For occasional use, in recommended doses, they're fine, and are often prescribed by natural healers for a wide range of complaints, including bladder ailments. In excess, diuretics can alter the body's electrolyte balance, which can be very dangerous. (Dandelion is the exception—it is rich in potassium, a mineral that is washed out of the body with most other diuretics.) Herbal diuretics are weaker and, therefore, safer than the synthetic diuretics that are prescribed to treat high blood pressure and other medical conditions. Nevertheless, I wouldn't use them constantly. As a weight loss tool, they are ineffective. Yes, you may lose a pound or two after taking them, but the results are only temporary. First, your body will compensate by making you thirstier and, therefore, you will drink more. Second, if overused, diuretics become ineffective. Your body needs water to survive and, in fact, if you don't drink enough water, it can interfere with your physical performance. So, you may be paying a very high price for vanity.

By the way, bloating and fluid retention should be checked by a doctor because it could be a sign of a more serious problem. Don't self-medicate!

If bloating is a problem, try cutting down on salty food to reduce water retention. If you are an endurance athlete, however, and are going to be exercising outdoors in the heat, don't eliminate salt from your diet. You need it to hold onto fluid to prevent your body from becoming overheated.

Possible Benefits

Helps you get rid of excess water weight.

How to Use It

Natural diuretics should be used only occasionally. Follow the directions on the package, and do not exceed recommended doses.

Cautions

People with kidney problems should avoid diuretics in general—unless prescribed by a physician—and potassium supplements or potassium-rich foods.

••

DMAE

••

2-dimethylaminoethanol (DMAE) is a smart drug that is reputed to improve mood and enhance memory. DMAE may increase levels of *acetylcholine*, a neurotransmitter in the brain. In order to understand how DMAE may work, you need to know a bit about your brain. Your brain consists of billions of specialized cells, called *neurons*. Brain cells communicate with each via a vast network of tiny branchlike connections, called *dendrites*. The dendrites never touch each other; nerve impulses are carried from one neuron to the other by releasing chemicals, called *neurotransmitters*. Neurotransmitters are the oil that keeps the brain running smoothly but, as we age, there is a decline in the production of neurotransmitters. Production of acetylcholine peaks at around age forty, then begins to gradually fall off. At any age, people with Alzheimer's disease have a severe shortage of acetylcholine, although it is not known whether this is the cause or the result of this debilitating ailment.

Acetylcholine is particularly important for memory and intellect. When levels of acetylcholine drop, it marks the beginning of age-related memory loss. Of course, there are other factors that contribute to the decline in mental function, including a drop in hormones such as DHEA, estrogen, and testosterone. However, since DMAE is a source of *choline*, the building block of acetylcholine, it makes sense that it can help reverse this mental decline.

DMAE has not been thoroughly studied on healthy people, but it has been tested as a treatment for Alzheimer's disease. The results have been mixed. In one uncontrolled study of senile patients, DMAE did not improve memory, but did improve mood and behavior. Personally, I think once the brain has deteriorated to such an advanced degree, there is little that can help it. It's my hope that protecting your brain (with the right lifestyle and supplements) will help prevent severe problems in brain function down the road.

Remember when your mom told you that fish was good for your brain? Sardines and anchovies are a rich source of DMAE!

Possible Benefits

May enhance memory.
Mood booster.

How to Use It

Take one to three 75 mg. tablets daily.

Cautions

DMAE should not be used by people with a history of epilepsy or convulsions. Some people find that DMAE causes especially vivid dreams.

EPHEDRA

Ephedra is one of those supplements that really gets a rise out of people. Some love it. Some hate it. Some want it banned. Others see the government's attempt to control it as nothing short of a conspiracy. Supporters of ephedra point out that it's been used in Chinese medicine for five thousand years. That's true, but not like it's being used (and maybe abused) today. In Asian medicine, ephedra is a traditional remedy for respiratory infections. It is only prescribed as an occasional treatment, not one to be used every day. In the West today, ephedra is the *hot* weight-loss supplement—even hotter when it's combined with caffeine and aspirin—the so-called

ECA stack. It is the primary ingredient of top-selling diet supplements like Metabolife. It is being marketed as a panacea for obesity, as well as a tool for body builders who want to squeeze out every ounce of body fat.

Ephedra, known in Chinese as *ma huang*, contains the amphetaminelike substances, ephedrine and pseudoephredine. Sound familiar? That's because these chemicals are common ingredients in cold medicines. You know how some antihistamines can make you jumpy? If taken in excess, ephredra can have the same effect.

The same chemicals that make you jumpy can also jumpstart your metabolism. Several studies have confirmed that, when compared to a placebo, ephedra can help obese people lose more weight—not a great deal more, but extra pounds, nonetheless. However, when combined with caffeine, ephedra works even better. In a study published in the *International Journal of Obesity*, 180 obese people were put on a weight-loss diet and given either ephedra alone, ephedra with caffeine, caffeine alone, or a placebo. At the end of twenty-four weeks, all the patients lost weight. Those taking ephedra plus caffeine lost 17.5 percent of their body weight; the ephedra alone lost 15.3 percent of body weight; caffeine alone lost 13.1 percent body weight, and the placebo group lost 13.5 percent. Obviously, those taking ephedra plus caffeine lost the most percentage of body weight. The researchers concluded, "The major finding of this drug study indicates that a combination of ephedrine (20 mg) + caffeine (200 mg) taken 3 times a day as an adjuvant to a low calorie diet improves weight loss. . . . The side effects such as tremor, tachycardia (heart palpitations) and insomnia are temporary. We found no serious withdrawal symptoms."

There's no dispute that ephedra speeds up metabolism, which promotes fat burning and weight loss. However, the patients taking placebos while dieting lost quite a bit of weight, too! And, when it comes down to actual pounds lost, the difference between the ephedra/caffeine users and placebo takers is not that great. For example, if someone began the regimen weighing two hundred pounds, they would have lost thirty-five pounds taking the ephedra/caffeine supplement, which is impressive. However, they would have lost twenty-seven pounds just by dieting! Of course, the more overweight you are, the more this gap grows. In my opinion, using strong medicine like ephedra may be useful for the very obese, but certainly not worth the risk for the run-of-the-mill "I've got to lose ten pounds" dieter.

The question is, is ephedra safe? As with any stimulant, ephedra can raise blood pressure, and cause irregular heart beat, insomnia, and headaches. According to the FDA, since 1994, some eight hundred people reported serious side effects, including death, from ephedra use. However, the Government Accounting Office recently rejected the FDA's attempt to put restrictions on ephedra, saying there wasn't enough scientific evidence to ban it. The fact is, ephedra is probably reasonably safe for most people if used cautiously and appropriately. By that I mean, if taken in the right doses by the right people. (Although sold in higher doses, the FDA does not recommend taking more than 24 mg. ephedra in a twenty-four-hour period for more than seven days.) Ephedra should not be used by anyone with high blood pressure, a heart condition, thyroid condition, diabetes, or anyone who is extremely sensitive to stimulants. Frankly, I think if you use ephedra, it should be under the supervision of a trained health-care practitioner with a knowledge of herbal supplements. You need to be carefully monitored to make sure that there are no untoward side effects. Women take note! The symptoms of heart disease are often overlooked in women so, before you use ephedra, be sure to be checked by a doctor who is familiar with this problem.

Kids have been known to take high doses of ephedra to get high. This is as stupid as it is dangerous. I dispute claims that ephedra is dangerous at low doses but, at high doses, I heartily agree it can be addictive and deadly.

Possible Benefits

Promotes weight loss.
Stimulant.

How to Use It

Do not exceed more than 24 mg. daily. Do not take too close to bedtime; it could keep you up. Do not use for more than one week.

ESSENTIAL FATTY ACIDS

 Low-fat diets have become a way of life for many Americans, who have been led to believe that cutting back on fat will save them from cancer, obesity, and heart disease. However, a diet too low in the right kinds of fat could be sabotaging your workout!

Essential fatty acids are essential nutrients that your body cannot produce by itself, and must obtain through food or supplements. Essential fatty acids are needed everywhere in the body. They are the major components of cell membranes. And hormones—the chemical messengers that run every body system—cannot be produced without them.

The body uses two types of essential fatty acids: omega 6 and omega 3. Some omega-3 fatty acids are converted in the body into eicosapentaenoic acid (EPA) and docosahexanoic acid (DHA). Both EPA and DHA are very important for physical and emotional health. A terrific immune booster, EPA increases natural killer-cell activity while decreasing prostaglandins, the hormonelike substances that promote inflammation. Low levels of DHA have been linked to depression, alcoholism, and violent behavior. Several test-tube studies have shown that omega-3 fatty acids can shrink cancerous tumors, and preliminary human studies suggest that these fats may have a potent inhibitory effect on breast cancer cells. Omega-3 fatty acids can also reduce high blood cholesterol and triglyceride levels.

There is also tantalizing new evidence that essential fatty acids may be effective for the inflammatory joint injuries commonly known as *tennis elbow* and *golf elbow*. A physiotherapist with Denmark's Olympic Committee reported that he has successfully treated hundreds of cases of recurrent inflammatory injuries with a combination of essential fatty acids and antioxidants, specifically omega-3 oil, omega-6 oil (from borage oil), and vitamins A, B6, C, E, plus selenium and zinc. The treatment was tested on rowers with Denmark's national rowing team. It took about two to three weeks for the athletes to respond to treatment, and those with severe injuries required more time, but the results were overwhelmingly positive. In fact, according to the researcher conducting the study, the combination of essential fatty acids and antioxidants may prove to be as effective as NSAIDS, but without the side effects, which include stomach distress and ulcers. Essential fatty acids boost the body's production of two beneficial hormonelike substances, type 1 and type 3 prostaglandins, which help soothe pain and inflammation.

Although there have been claims that essential fatty acids build muscle, there is no scientific evidence to back this up. This is not to say that essential fatty acids are not required to maintain lean body mass. I believe they are, however, the mechanism by which they work has not yet been discovered. Animal studies suggest that essential fatty acids may reduce the damaging effects of the stress hormone *cortisol*, which is one way they could help retain muscle. When the body is under extreme stress (like when you're really working it hard), your adrenal glands pump stress hormones to give you added energy. The problem is that these hormones also break down muscle as fuel. So, sometimes, the harder you work, the less you gain! A recent Israeli study published in the *International Journal of Neuroscience* reported that essential fatty acids helped block the damaging effects of cortisol on brain cells in rats. In particular, the stressed-out rats given essential fatty acids performed better on tests that required memory and concentration than stressed-out rats not given essential fatty acids. What's exciting about this finding is the possibility that essential fatty acids may protect humans against cortisol damage, not just in the brain, but other parts of the body as well.

Possible Benefits

Promotes healing of sports injuries.
Reduces pain and inflammation.
Counters the harmful effects of cortisol.

How to Use It

Take an essential fatty acid supplement containing 2000 mg. omega-3 fatty acids, consisting of 360 mg. EPA and 240 mg. DHA, plus 90 mg. GLA.

ESTROGEN BLOCKERS

Estrogen blockers are supplements that inhibit the action of potent estrogens in both men and women. These supplements include DIM, ipriflavone, and chrysin. If you're a guy, you may be thinking, "Hey what am I doing with estrogen?" The fact is, both men and women produce estrogen and testosterone. Obviously, guys make a lot more testosterone, and women make more estrogen. Both hormones are necessary for normal physical and mental function. Paradoxically, estrogen blockers are weaker forms of estrogens found in plants called phytoestrogens. For men, estrogen blockers inhibit an enzyme that converts testosterone into *estradiol*, a potent estrogen that can stimulate the growth of hormone-sensitive cancers (like in the prostate). As men age, they make more of this enzyme, which not only increases their risk of developing cancer, but leaves them less testosterone for muscle and strength. Men at any age who take excessive prohormones like andro and DHEA to boost their testosterone levels may inadvertently end up with more estradiol than they bargained for. The same is true for men who use prescription testosterone. The side effects of too much estrogen in men can be downright embarrassing. (Remember that great cartoon of Mark McGwire in a bra?) Some supplement manufacturers claim that, if you take estrogen blockers, you can take prohormones such as andro and DHEA without having to worry about the estrogen problem. I haven't seen any studies to convince me that this is true. Frankly, I think if you mess around with hormones, you need to do so carefully. And whether you choose to use estrogen blockers or not, you should have your hormone levels monitored by a doctor.

For women, estrogen blockers also reduce the production of *estradiol*, a strong estrogen which may be linked to an increased risk of breast cancer. In premenopausal women, they bind to estrogen receptors on cells and trick the cells into believing that there is no need to produce more estrogen. In postmenopausal women, they take the place of estrogen, and may relieve many of the symptoms of menopause, as well as help stem bone loss that can lead to osteoporosis.

Possible Benefits

May block the production of potent estrogens.

May reduce the risk of cancer.

May help maintain testosterone levels in older men.

How to Use It

Doses vary according to product. Take as directed on the package.

FAT BLOCKERS

Fat blockers are supplements—chitosan and chitin are the best known—that inhibit the absorption of fat by the digestive tract. *Chitosan* (which is a form of processed chitin) is a type of fiber derived from the shells of shellfish. It binds to fat and flushes it out of your system. Natural fat blockers are similar in action to the stronger prescription fat blockers like Xenical. Chitosan, often in combination with other forms of fiber, is promoted as a weight-loss product. Numerous studies confirm that it can lower high cholesterol levels and may even have antioxidant activity.

People frequently ask me, "If I take fat blockers with my meals, does that mean that I can eat all I want without gaining weight?" My answer is always an emphatic *no!* Fat blockers are not a cure for poor eating habits or obesity. If you eat a high-fat diet, fat blockers are not going to make you thin. Fat blockers can eliminate some, but not all, fat. Fat is more fattening than protein or carbohydrates (one gram of fat is nine calories, versus four calories for one gram of protein or carbohydrate) so eating a lot of fat is going to put pounds on you. If you want to lose weight and keep it off, the only solution is to change your eating habits, and that means limiting your intake of fatty foods. There's another problem with fat blockers—they may also rid your body of good things, like fat-soluble vitamins, minerals, and other nutrients. Animal studies have shown that chitosan can interfere with the absorption of other nutrients. In fact, if you take these products, you must take a vitamin and mineral supplement to replenish what you may be losing. Finally, fat blockers don't discriminate between good fats and bad fats.

Our bodies need essential fatty acids to function well, and fat blockers may target these good fats as zealously as bad fats.

Nevertheless, despite my reservations, fat blockers may be a useful tool in helping you jumpstart a weight-loss program, but they should be taken along with a sensible eating plan. Fat blockers may cause some unpleasant side effects—gas and stomach upset is one of them.

Human studies on chitosan have primarily focused on its role as a cholesterol-lowering agent. I could not find any major clinical trials confirming chitosan in which chitosan has been used effectively as a weight-loss tool.

Possible Benefits

By reducing fat absorption, may help in weight loss.
Can lower high cholesterol.

How to Use It

The usual dose is one to two 500 mg. capsules of chitosan or a fiber/fat-blocker combination before meals. Drink a full glass of water to avoid digestive discomfort.

Caution

Do not use this product if you have an intestinal condition, or a problem absorbing nutrients, without consulting your physician.

FLAVONOIDS

Better sex, better mental focus, better health. That's the promise of *flavonoids*, a group of more than four thousand individual compounds found primarily in the pigments of leaves, barks, rinds, seeds, and flowers. About fifty flavonoids are present in foods and beverages derived from plants, such as berries, tea, and wine. Flavonoids, which are powerful antioxidants, enhance the activity of vitamin C in the body. These remarkable phytochemicals also appear to reduce the risk of cancer and heart disease. They are truly deserving of their spot on my hot hundred list

Flavonoids are found in ginkgo, grape-seed extract, pine-bark extract as well as on blueberries, cranberries, apples, onions, and citrus fruit. Flavonoids play many roles in the body, but perhaps the most important is that they regulate nitric oxide (NO). NO is a colorless gas produced by many different cells that, among other things, helps modulate communication between brain cells, which is important for thinking and learning. Too much or too little nitric oxide can have a devastating effect on the body. Flavonoids help maintain nitric oxide within a beneficial range. Flavonoids also improve the circulation of blood throughout the body, including the brain, which gets oxygen and nutrients from blood. Not surprisingly, flavonoids are often touted as brain boosters. Some alternative physicians have even reported success in using flavonoids to treat patients with attention deficit hyperactivity disorder (ADHD).

The ability to control nitric oxide and improve circulation also make flavonoids a sex-enhancing supplement. The right level of nitric oxide is key to achieving and maintaining an erection—in fact, Viagra is also a nitric-oxide modulator. Perhaps even more important, however, is the fact that flavonoids can prevent arteries from becoming clogged, which interferes with blood flow. It may surprise you to learn that poor circulation due to atherosclerosis is the number one cause of erectile dysfunction in men. Taking flavonoids now could help prevent sexual problems later.

Here's more good news about flavonoids—they are terrific immune boosters. Be sure to take them during cold and flu season. By the way, they can even relieve allergy symptoms! So, if you're spending less time outdoors during the peak allergy season, include bioflavonoids in your supplement regimen.

Possible Benefits

Improve mental function and concentration.
May improve sexual function.
Helps prevent infection.
Good for the heart.

How to Use It

Take 2500 mg. mixed citrus bioflavonoids daily. Specialty flavonoids such as ginkgo and PCOs are more expensive, and may be more effective for particular problems, such as age-related memory impairment. However, for most people, citrus bioflavonoids will be enough.

FORSKOLIN

facts Forskolin, an extract from the *Coleus forskohlii* plant, is another ancient Ayurvedic herb from the Indian traditional system of medicine that has found its way to the modern-day gym. It is usually not taken as a single herb; it is incorporated in fitness formulas specifically designed to burn fat and increase metabolism. Forskolin turns on the adenylate cyclase enzyme, which boosts levels of another chemical, cyclic adenosine monophosphate (cAMP) in cells. This triggers a cascade of events that increases the release and production of thyroid hormone, which raises metabolism. The higher the metabolic rate, the faster fat is burned for energy.

For centuries, the *Coleus forskohlii* plant has been used to treat a wide range of ailments, including high blood pressure, eczema, asthma, and allergies. Alternative physicians prescribe *Coleus forskohlii* for many heart conditions. If you have heart disease or high blood pressure, do not use this herb unless it is under a doctor's supervision.

Forskolin is also good for some digestive problems, particularly those related to sluggish production of stomach acid. In fact, as people age, one of the leading causes of indigestion is a decline in the production of hydrochloric acid, or HCL, which is essential for the breakdown of proteins. Forskolin increases the secretion of HCL and other digestive enzymes, which helps improve the breakdown and absorption of food. However, if you have ulcers, avoid this herb—you don't need the additional acid!

Studies performed in India suggest that forskolin may also have anticancer activity. It inhibits the growth of tumors in animals injected with cancerous cells and appears to stimulate immune system activity.

Possible Benefits

Speeds up metabolism.
Heart healthy.

Helps digestion.

Cancer fighter.

How to Use It

Take one to three 250 mg. capsules daily.

Caution

If you're taking any prescription medicine (antidepressants, antihistamines), check with your physician before using this herb. Forskolin may be included in supplements designed for fat burning; be sure to look over the ingredients before using these products.

GAMMA ORYZANOL

 Gamma oryzanol is one of the many sports supplements that highlight the fact that there is a crying need for more human studies. Gamma oryzanol, a natural component of rice bran, is a mixture of *plant sterols* (hormonelike substances) and ferulic acid. First used in Japan, gamma oyrzanol was introduced in the United States in the late 1980s for human and animal use. This stuff looks interesting, and may work well as an ergonomic aid and muscle builder, but there are no controlled studies to verify the anecdotal data. Despite the lack of science, gamma oryzanol has attracted a steady following of body builders who claim it works well for them. There are others, however, who say it doesn't do anything! So, if you're interested, I guess it falls into the try-it-yourself-and-see-if-it-works category.

What's really intriguing is the fact that gamma oryzanol is used as a peak performance supplement for *racehorses*. According to *Michael Plumb's Horse Journal* gamma oryzanol can give horses bigger muscles. Despite rigorous training schedules, horses maintained their stamina and concentration.

Okay, so gamma oryzanol may make horses better athletes. Does it work for humans? In one small study of trained weight lifters, gamma orzyanol increased body weight significantly more than a placebo, and increased body strength in one out of three measures. In a larger study, however, it did nothing. It would be nice if there were more double-blind, placebo-controlled studies to refer you to, but if there are any, I can't find them! Manufacturers of gamma oryzanol will provide testimonials from happy clients who claim that gamma oryzanol changed their physique, but take these with a grain of salt. Chances are, these guys are also doing lots of other stuff that could be contributing to their physical transformation, like intense exercise, eating the right diet, and or taking other supplements.

Two other studies conducted on gamma oryzanol have suggested it could be a valuable aid for menopausal women. In the 1960s, Japanese researchers tested gamma oryzanol on women who had surgical hysterectomies that induced menopause. They found that gamma oryzanol worked exceptionally well in relieving symptoms like hot flashes. It also helped reduce high cholesterol and triglyceride levels and boosted the levels of HDL, or good cholesterol. Gamma oryzanol is also an antioxidant, which means it protects against those nasty free radicals that can make it harder for you to recover from your workout, and age you prematurely.

Possible Benefits

May build muscle (in humans and horses).
Helps normalize cholesterol.
Relieves menopausal symptoms.

How to Use It

Look for the soluble, liquid form. Take 1 teaspoon daily (about 330 mg.) per one hundred pounds of body weight.

GINKGO

When I first wrote about gingko biloba (the preferred form of ginkgo) in the *Herb Bible* a decade ago, few people knew what it was and even fewer could pronounce it.

Today, it has become one of the best-selling supplements of all time. There are commercials for it on television, and recently, several manufacturers have put it in snack food! No wonder it's so popular—it's being touted as the supplement that can make you smarter and sexier. Actually, ginkgo is nothing new—it's been used for more than five thousand years in traditional Chinese medicine. Only recently have scientists learned how ginkgo works—it's an antioxidant and anti-inflammatory. Gingko improves the flow of blood throughout the body. In fact, it's ability to boost mental function has been attributed to improved circulation to the brain. The antioxidants in gingko, however, may also protect the brain against further damage by free radicals, a major factor in brain aging. The same antioxidants may help speed recovery after your workout, and protect against muscle damage.

It may surprise you to learn that the major cause of erectile dysfunction (impotence) is poor circulation due to atherosclerosis, or clogged arteries. In order to achieve an erection, you need to have enough blood flowing to the penis. Since gingko helps improve blood flow, researchers tested it on men suffering from erectile problems. Some men in the study were also given injections of a drug called papaverine, a muscle stimulant that can enhance erections. The men using gingko alone or the gingko papaverine combination showed great improvement in erections. So . . . for guys who have an occasional problem, gingko may do the trick.

Will ginkgo really make you smarter? Recently, an extract of ginkgo was found to alter brain waves in a positive way in healthy people, which suggested that ginkgo extract could improve concentration and memory. A few studies—primarily performed in Europe where ginkgo is widely prescribed—have confirmed that this herb can speed reaction time and improve short-term memory in healthy people. I know from personal experience that gingko makes you more alert. In fact, some people find that if they take ginkgo late in the day, it can cause insomnia. A much-publicized study conducted at the New York Institute for Medical Research on patients suffering from dementia (either due to stroke or Alzheimer's disease) showed that daily ginkgo supplements improved performance on tests measuring cognitive ability and memory better than a placebo in 30 percent of the subjects. Other studies have yielded similar results. The National Center for Complementary and Alternative Medicine and the National Institute on Aging are funding a six-year study at the University of Pittsburgh Medical School to determine whether taking gingko before you show signs of brain aging could prevent or delay the onset of dementia. Frankly, I think the earlier you begin taking care of your brain, the longer you will keep it in peak condition.

Ginkgo is also a natural blood thinner, which means it protects against blood clots. However, if you're having surgery, do tell your physician that you are taking ginkgo. You may have to discontinue it a week or so prior to surgery. If you're using gingko with other blood thinners, like coumadin or aspirin, be sure to tell your doctor so that your medication can be adjusted accordingly, and that you can be monitored.

Possible Benefits

Sharpens your brain.

Improves sexual function in men.

Good antioxidant.

How to Use It

Take two 60 mg. ginkgo biloba tablets daily. Although ginkgo is often included in chips and snack bars, there's not very much of it.

GINSENG

Ginseng refers to several different types of plants, not all related, that are purported to boost energy, increase stamina, and help the body better withstand stress, among other health benefits. Soviet scientists called ginseng an *adaptogen* because they believed it helps people adapt to new challenges, like an increased exercise load, a change in outdoor temperature, or emotional stress. For thousands of years, ginseng has been a staple of the traditional Asian pharmacy. Modern scientists have confirmed that ginseng can boost immune function and, according to animal studies, may even reduce the risk of several different cancers. A recent British study showed the just one dose of ginseng can speed reaction time and improve memory and concentration. What is less known is whether or not ginseng can actually improve *physical* performance.

For those of you unfamiliar with ginseng, let me tell you a bit about the different varieties. There are three primary types of ginseng on the market in the United States: American ginseng, Asian ginseng, and Siberian ginseng, also called *ciwujia*, which is not actually a member of the ginseng family, but a related plant that offers many of the same benefits. To clear up some of the confusion, true members of the ginseng family all have the word *Panax* (Greek for cure all) in their scientific name. For example, Asian ginseng is *Panax ginseng;* American ginseng is *Panax quinquefolium.* Siberian ginseng, however, is *Eleutherococcus senticosus.* Asian ginseng is reputed to be the most potent; American ginseng the mildest. Siberian ginseng is considered the best for stress-related problems. Although ginseng is one of the top ten herbs purchased in the United States—Americans spend $86 million on ginseng annually—there is no guarantee that the ginseng you are buying is any good. Many products are so watered down that they are ineffective. In fact, a recent analysis of fifty-four ginseng products found that 60 percent were worthless and 25 percent did not contain any ginseng. Only buy ginseng from reputable companies that guarantee the strength and potency of their products.

Some athletes swear that ginseng gives them the competitive edge, but researchers have not been able to back up these claims in clinical studies. Unfortunately, there are few reliable studies. A recent double-blind study of thirty-one men who took either Asian ginseng capsules or a placebo for eight weeks did not show any improvement in performance or stamina between the two groups. I believe that ginseng's affect on athletic performance may not be due to its physical impact, but rather, its effect on mental function. Several studies have documented that ginseng improves concentration and boosts mood. In fact, a recent study of two thousand people showed that a standardized extract of ginseng along with a multivitamin and minerals produced a reduction in fatigue, and increased feelings of well-being. When you're working out hard, or trying to run the last mile in a marathon, having a clear head and a strong focus can be the difference between success or failure.

Ginseng may improve your performance in the bedroom. Studies have shown that it improves sperm count, and raises testosterone plasma levels. In fact, a recent study of men with erectile dysfunction found that ginseng helped improve sexual function, while enhancing libido. Interestingly, *ginsenoides*, the active chemical ingredients in ginseng, are very similar in structure to steroid hormones.

Although the medical establishment remains suspicious of natural products like ginseng, the German Commission E, the equivalent of our FDA, has recommended ginseng as a "tonic for invigoration and fortification in times of fatigue and debility or declining capacity for work and concentration also during convalescence."

Possible Benefits

Improves immune function.
Increases mental energy.
Reputed to enhance physical stamina.
May boost sexual function.

How to Use It

Ginsenosides are the active ingredients in ginseng: Look for products that contain 10 percent ginsenosides. The usual dose is two to three capsules daily. Start with a lower dose to see if ginseng makes you jittery.

Cautions

In comparison to other natural products, ginseng has been thoroughly studied in terms of its potential side effects with other medications. People with heart problems or high blood pressure should check with their health practitioner before using ginseng. If you are taking corticosteroids, ginseng may enhance the effect of these drugs. If you have diabetes or insulin resistance, be sure to have your blood-sugar levels monitored carefully if you use ginseng; it could have an additional hypoglycemic effect. Do not use in combination with monoamine oxidase inhibitors (MAOIs); it could cause increased agitation. If you use ginseng, don't overdo the caffeine. Ginseng may cause breast tenderness in some women because it contains phytoestrogens. In rare cases, it may cause vaginal bleeding in menopausal women.

GLUCOMANNAN

 Glucomannan is a powder made from the tuber of a plant known in the West as *Devil's Tongue* and in Japan as *Konhac* or *konnyaku*. In Japan, glucocomannan is used as flour to make noodles or added to stews and sauces as a thickening agent. Unlike the refined white flour used in the West, glucomannan is rich in nutrients and high in soluble fiber. Because it is so high in fiber, it helps speed food through the intestinal tract, which has given it a reputation as a weight-loss supplement. In particular, glucomannan is reputed to decrease the absorption of dietary fats, which would, of course, help weight loss. Like other types of fiber, glucomannan expands in the stomach, creating a feeling of fullness. The Japanese claim that glucomannan helps keep them slim, but their typical vegetable-based, low-fat Asian diet probably plays an even more important role. I view glucomannan as a useful tool that could enhance the effects of an overall weight-reduction program, which includes smart eating and exercise. Frankly, I don't think that it (or anything else) will work alone.

Glucomannan can reduce high cholesterol levels, specifically lowering bad cholesterol, LDL. In animal studies it's been shown to help maintain normal glucose levels, which may make it a useful adjuvant therapy for Type II (adult onset) diabetes. This shouldn't be surprising—a high-fiber diet is often prescribed for people with Type II diabetes. In fact, if people ate more fiber, less fat, and less junk carbohydrates (like soda, cookies, and chips), I have no doubt that the epidemic of adult onset diabetes could be reversed. (If you have diabetes of any type, please seek treatment from a nutritionally oriented physician.)

If you use glucomannan, you may also be losing some fat-soluble vitamins (like E, A, and carotenoids) along with the fat, so please be sure to take your supplements.

Glucomannan appears to increase the amount of good bacteria in the gut, which can help protect against cancer.

Possible Benefits

Good source of fiber.
Interferes with the absorption of fat.
Normalizes blood sugar.

How to Use It

The usual dose is one to two 500–700 mg. capsules before meals. Take with a full glass of water to avoid stomach distress.

Cautions

If you have gastrointestinal problems (like gasiness or problems with food absorption), do not use this product without consulting with your physician.

GLUCOSAMINE

Glucosamine is a naturally occurring substance found in all human tissue, but in highest concentrations in *articular cartilage*, the thin coating that allows joints to move with fluidity. Glusosamine is well known as one of two supplements of the so-called arthritis cure. (The other supplement is chondroitin, page 50.) You may be tempted not to read this section because you think, "I'm young and strong; why worry about arthritis?" but you'd be making a serious mistake. At any age, if you train hard, you need to know about this supplement. If you're forty plus, you probably should be taking it.

The wearing away of articular cartilage, either through traumatic injury or overuse, can result in osteoarthritis. Although joint illnesses such as osteoarthritis and bone pain are the most common illnesses of aging, by age thirty, 50 percent of all people are affected by degenerative joint changes. The most common causes are chronic stress and strain, for example, from competitive sports, or work-related injuries. Weight lifters beware: Carrying heavy loads increases the risk of osteoarthritis.

Several have documented that glucosamine can relieve the pain and stiffness of osteoarthritis as well as NSAIDs. In a randomized double-blind-placebo controlled study, patients with osteoarthritis of the knee were given 1.5 grams of glucosamine sulfate daily or 1.2 grams of ibuprofen. Although the ibuprofen worked faster, by the eighth week of treatment, there was no difference in pain relief among both groups. So, why not take ibuprofen if it works faster? NSAIDs like ibuprofen can not only cause serious side effects including stomach bleeding, but can cause further destruction of the joint. Glucosamine not only reduces pain, but may also trigger the regeneration of cartilage. In fact, a new three-year study of patients with osteoarthritis of the knee shows that glucosamine not only significantly reduced arthritic symptoms compared to a placebo, but seemed to improve the overall condition of the knee joint. In other words, glucosamine appeared to stop and even reverse the degenerative process. The earlier you take glucosamine, the better. Glusosamine can only help regenerate cartilage if there are still functioning *chondrocytes*, cartilage-producing cells. If you wait too long, it won't work.

Glucosamine may also help promote the healing of overuse injuries, which, as noted earlier, can put you on the fast track for osteoarthritis. If you are recovering from an injury, I suggest that you try glucosamine—it may speed up your recovery. The best advice I can give, however, is to avoid activities that severely overtax your joints. You may think that you're making yourself stronger but, in reality, a severe injury can take you out of the game altogether.

A word to weekend athletes: You are especially prone to joint injuries because you try to pack a full week's worth of activities into one or two days. Take it easy! Be meticulous about warming up your muscles before exercise. Muscles support your joints and, if your muscles aren't working properly, your joints will suffer. Do strengthening exercises during the week to keep yourself in shape for your weekend. Thirty minutes of resistance training twice a week can make a huge difference in muscle strength, and spare you from weekend-warrior battle scars.

Don't even dream about doing activities like skiing if you're out of shape—the risk of injury is too great. Keep in mind that today's injury could be tomorrow's osteoarthritis.

Can taking glucosamine prevent osteoarthritis down the road? Some experts believe that it can, especially since it helps maintain cartilage, but there are no studies yet to prove this.

Possible Benefits

Relieves pain and stiffness of osteoarthritis.
Promotes healing of joints.

How to Use It

Take up to three 500 mg. tablets daily.

GLUTAMINE

facts *Amino acids* are the building blocks of protein and, of them, glutamine is the most abundant. *Glutamine* comprises more than half of the total amount of amino acids within the body and 60 percent of the total amino acids within muscle. Glutamine is a nonessential amino acid because it is made by the body and not obtained through food. The theory is that the body makes enough glutamine to meet the needs of most people. But, if you work out hard, or participate in endurance sports, I can guarantee you that glutamine supplementation *is* essential for your health.

Glutamine is a substrate of *glutathione*, the body's primary antioxidant, which means it is a necessary ingredient for the production of glutathione. When you work your body hard, you are depleting it of glutathione. Low levels of glutathione are a harbinger of illness—keep your levels of glutathione high!

Among its many roles in the body, glutamine helps replenish *glycogen*, the principle form in which carbohydrate is stored in the liver and the muscles. As the body needs it, glycogen can be quickly converted into *glucose*, an important source of energy. Remember, if you don't have enough glycogen on hand, your body will begin breaking down lean tissue, which will hamper your ability to build muscle. Glutamine is also important for muscle repair and has been used to treat wasting syndrome in patients confined to long periods of bed rest.

Glutamine is not only good for muscle, but appears to have a powerful effect on the immune system. In fact, it has been dubbed "fuel for immune cells." Earlier, I pointed out that endurance athletes are especially vulnerable to upper-respiratory-tract infections after prolonged training or competition. The measurable decline in immune-cell activity after severe physical exertion can last for days. There are several reasons for this. First, during intense exercise, the body consumes oxygen at a much higher rate. High oxygen use leads to more free radicals which in turn, depletes immune-boosting antioxidants. Second, although glutamine levels rise after moderate physical activity, they plummet after intense exercise. When the body is under physical stress, it quickly depletes its store of glutamine. Several studies have reported that glutamine supplements reduce the incidence of infections reported by athletes after strenuous physical activity. Glutamine also helped the athlete's immune system recover more quickly after exertion.

Glutamine can inhibit the biochemical reaction that leads to sugar highs and lows, which trigger food cravings and overeating. Glutamine is essential to maintain a steady stream of glucose, the fuel used by the brain. If you're having difficulty concentrating, or find that you are feeling low at various points in the day, glutamine may be just what you need to keep your energy levels stable.

If you frequently take NSAIDs to help relieve post-workout aches and pains, you know that you are risking injury to your stomach lining. The good news is that the same supplement that is helping to maintain muscle and keep you healthy may also prevent NSAID-related damage in your gut. German scientists recently reported that glutamine has a protective effect on the lining of the gut. They found that it can help preserve the integrity of the mucosal cells of the intestines during radiation and chemotherapy which, under the best of circumstances, can often cause damage to healthy tissues and organs.

Possible Benefits

Essential for preserving muscle.
Energizes the body and the mind.

Helps prevent exercise-related decline in immunity.

Speeds up post-workout recovery.

How to Use It

Glutamine is usually sold in the form of L-glutamine. (L- before an amino acid refers to its chemical structure.) L-glutamine is available in powder, which is the most economical form. Mix 1 teaspoon L-glutamine in liquid. Drink up to one hour before and immediately following your workout. If you are sick, increase your dose to three teaspoons of L-glutamine daily.

GLUTATHIONE

Glutathione has been dubbed nature's master antioxidant, because of the many vital roles it plays in the body. Glutathione is the primary antioxidant in your cells. In fact, glutathione is so important that low levels put you at risk of disease, premature aging, and death. Levels of glutathione decline with age. During times of illness or stress, your levels of glutathione will plummet. If you train hard, beware! Studies performed by Dr. Lester Packer, Ph.D., of the world renowned Packer Lab at the University of California at Berkeley have shown that levels of glutathione can be seriously depleted by strenuous exercise.

The impact of glutathione depletion is felt almost immediately, even by the most fit. As noted earlier, marathon runners often contract a respiratory infection immediately following a big race. Numerous studies have shown that glutathione depletion can seriously hamper the ability of immune cells to do their job, thereby leaving the body vulnerable to every bug that comes its way.

Glutathione depletion will also hurt you in the long run. There is a high concentration of glutathione in the liver. One of the liver's primary jobs is to detoxify drugs and poisons that may be ingested in food, drugs, or produced by the body through normal metabolism. Glutathione plays an important part in the detoxification process. If you don't have enough glutathione, you increase your exposure to toxins.

Steroid hormones (like testosterone and estrogen) are also broken down in the liver. Numerous studies suggest that higher than normal levels of steroid hormones can cause serious problems, such as cancer. Since glutathione helps maintain normal hormone levels, if you are taking supplements that boost testosterone, it is even more critical for you be mindful of your glutathione levels. Glutathione also helps to control chronic inflammation, which can lead to arthritis, heart disease, and cancer.

Glutathione is also involved in the storage and transport of amino acids, the building blocks of protein. Without adequate amounts of protein, you can't maintain or repair muscle and, without glutathione, you can't make protein.

Glutathione is available as a supplement, but you should know that there is some controversy as to whether or not it can be absorbed digestively. Many scientists believe that only small amounts of glutathione can pass from the gastrointestinal tract to the bloodstream, and therefore, very high doses are needed to have any effect. Interestingly, you may be able to raise your glutathione levels more efficiently by taking two other supplements, lipoic acid (page 115) (alpha lipoic acid) and NAC (page 122). Studies have shown that both of these supplements can increase blood levels of glutathione. Glutathione is abundant in fruits and vegetables so, if you eat a lot of these healthy foods, you are getting some glutathione.

Possible Benefits

Essential for life.
Boosts immune function.
Critical for detoxification process.

How to Use It

Since glutathione supplements are poorly absorbed by the body, the best way to raise your glutathione levels is to take lipoic acid (alpha lipoic acid) or NAC.

GLYCEROL

Every savvy athlete worries about *dehydration*, the excessive loss of body fluid. At the very least, dehydration can interfere with your ability to perform well. At the very worst, it can be life threatening. You lose fluid through sweat, breath, and urination. The harder you work out, the more fluid you are likely to lose. Even a small loss of fluid can hurt your game. Sixty-five percent of your body weight is fluid. Just a 3 percent drop in fluid can result in a 20 to 30 percent decline in performance! Severe dehydration can also result in heat exhaustion, shock, and death. Fortunately, most athletes can weather some dehydration without fatal consequences. However, it's important to know that if you push too hard, too often, you can get hurt.

The best way to handle dehydration is to prevent it from happening in the first place. A day or two before the event, be sure to drink at least eight glasses of water daily. Avoid caffeinated beverages and alcohol, diuretics that can accelerate fluid loss. Consider using glycerol, a metabolite of alcohol without any of alcohol's negative properties: It won't intoxicate or dehydrate you, but will help stem the loss of fluid during intense exercise. Glycerol is part of the body's citric acid cycle of aerobic-energy metabolism. It also increases the amount of water in muscle. It is included in many sports-performance beverages, and seems to work well, especially in warm weather. In a study conducted at the Veterans Affairs Medical Center in Albuquerque, N.M., athletes taking glycerol were able to exercise longer in the heat than those taking a placebo. In addition, the glycerol users had lower heart rates, which meant that there was more blood to send to the skin to cool it down, and to send to muscles for oxygen.

Possible Benefits

Helps prevent dehydration.
May improve athletic performance in warm weather.

How to Use It

Drink a glycerol-containing beverage one hour before an event. If you use glycerol, be sure to drink enough water. (Drink a few ounces every fifteen minutes.) If you don't drink enough water, glycerol could make you feel nauseated and headachey.

GREEN TEA

 Recently, when I traveled to Japan, I was amazed at the difference between the Japanese and American physique. Japanese tend to be slim and sleek. It is unusual to see an overweight person. In contrast, most Americans appear fat and flabby. Granted, there are real differences in the Asian diet *versus* the Western diet that may explain the difference in body type. Japanese eat more lean fish and vegetables, and less sweets, but I don't think that's the whole answer. A recent study published in the *Journal of Clinical Nutrition* suggests that the Japanese may owe their trim figures to their favorite beverage—green tea.

Green tea is the national beverage of Japan and is served at every meal. I have been writing about green tea for years. It has been studied extensively for its anticancer properties, and has been linked to a reduced risk of colon, breast, and lung cancer. It is well known that green tea can prevent the oxidation of LDL cholesterol (a process that increases the risk of having a heart attack) and contains natural antibacterial chemicals that fight tooth decay. Scientists have just uncovered something completely new about this traditional drink: Green tea contains a unique combination of phytochemicals that can help you lose weight! Like coffee, green tea contains caffeine, known to increase *thermogenesis*, the burning of fat. (Green tea contains only half as much caffeine as coffee.) Caffeine, however, is not the primary reason why green tea is being touted as a potential weight-loss aid. Rather, it is an antioxidant flavonoid in green tea called *epigallocatechin* (EGCG) that may hold the key to slimming. In a twenty-four-hour study designed to measure energy expenditure conducted at the University of Fribourg in Switzerland, researchers gave ten men two capsules of EGCG with each meal. On different days, they gave the men caffeine capsules or a placebo. While taking the green-tea capsules, the men increased over-all energy expenditure by 4 percent and fat burning by 10 percent more than those taking the caffeine capsules. That amounts to eighty additional calories daily which, over the course of a year, adds up to a savings of about 29,000 calories or eight and a half pounds. No one has studied whether drinking green tea will have the same effect, but I suspect that it does, though the effect will not be as dramatic as taking the supplements.

Unlike drugs used to lose weight, green-tea extract has no adverse side effects; in fact, there are only side benefits. The antioxidants are actually good for your body. So, here's one weight-loss supplement I can wholeheartedly recommend.

Possible Benefits

Helps turn up fat metabolism.
Can help shed extra pounds.
Protects against cancer and heart disease.

How to Use It

Steep one tea bag in boiling water for two minutes, or take two tablets of caffeine-free extract daily.

GUARANA

 Coffee, tea . . . or guarana. If you're looking for a caffeine charge, then guarana can do the job as well as other, better-known, caffeine sources. Straight from the Amazon, *guarana* is an herb that contains *guaranine*, a chemical that is a dead ringer for caffeine and its chemical cousins, theophylline and theobromine. Guarana is often promoted as an energizer but, frankly, I don't think it's the best herb for stamina and endurance. Caffeine gives you a quick spike of energy, but the effects are not long lasting.

Look for guarana in thermogenic formulas designed to turn up metabolism and burn fat. These fat-burning wonders often contain ephedra, white willow or aspirin, caffeine, kola, and other herbs. The problem is, like caffeine, a little guarana goes a long way. Too much can make you very jittery. Caffeine can also be unsafe for people with high blood pressure, heart disease, and other conditions. Having offered these caveats, the question that remains is whether guarana can help shed fat. There have not been a lot of studies using guarana instead of straight caffeine, but I suspect it works in a similar fashion. In fact, guarana is so similar to caffeine that I don't advise combining it with other caffeine-containing products, so that means limiting your intake of cola, coffee, tea, and chocolate. Also, if you are taking a metabolic enhancer, be sure that it doesn't combine different sources of caffeine.

Possible Benefits

Enhances the fat-burning effect of ephedra.
May give you a lift.

How to Use It

Take one 200 mg. capsule for an occasional lift, but not too often!

GUGGUL

Guggul, sometimes called *guggulipid*, is a yellowish resin produced by the stem of the Cammiphora Mukul plant of India. Guggul is part of the Ayurvedic system of traditional medicine. It has been used by Indian healers for thousands of years to treat heart disease, obesity, and arthritis. Several studies confirm that guggul can help reduce the levels of bad cholesterol and *triglycerides*, lipids that increase the risk of heart disease. At the same time, it increases the levels of good cholesterol (HDL), which cleans out the arteries.

Guggul is not only good for your heart—it may be good for your physique. Recently, guggul has been promoted as a supplement that can help burn fat. You will find it in many sports formulas designed to boost metabolism. Guggul appears to work by stimulating the thyroid gland, which increases the production of thyroid hormone. Thyroid hormone is critical for normal metabolism. A sluggish thyroid could contribute to excess weight gain and retention of fat. In one study, conducted in India, of obese people on a weight-loss diet, guggul users had significantly more weight loss than those who took a placebo. Given the fact that guggul has been used as a weight-reducing agent for thousands of years, I think it's worth a closer look.

Guggul is also an effective anti-inflammatory and can help relieve joint pain and inflammation.

The active ingredient in guggul are steroidlike chemicals called *guggul stones:* Most extracts contain 5 to 10 percent guggul stones.

Possible Benefits

Burns fat, may help weight loss.
Relieves symptoms of arthritis.

How to Use It

Take three 25 mg. capsules daily for twelve to twenty-four weeks.

Caution

People with liver disease or bowel disorders should not use guggul unless it is under the supervision of a physician.

HMB

 If I were designing the perfect muscle builder, it would have to meet several stringent criteria. First and foremost, it would increase muscle size and strength. Second, unlike some other muscle builders (particularly anabolic steroids and T-boosters), it must be completely safe for just about everyone. Third, because I'm so demanding about what I put in my body, it would offer other health benefits, such as protection against heart disease. And, while I'm dreaming, it would be great if the same supplement could put you in a good mood (as opposed to steroids, which can make you downright nasty). Well, folks, I think I've found a muscle builder that comes close to meeting all these requirements. It's *b-hydroxy-b-methybutyrate*

(HMB), a metabolite of the branched-chain amino-acid leucine. HMB is not a drug or chemical; it is naturally produced in the body from foods containing leucine. When taken as a supplement, however, the results can be dramatic.

Several human studies confirm that both men and women can benefit from HMB supplementation. Those who follow a strength-resistance training program who took on average 3 grams HMB daily had one and a half to two times the increase in strength and muscle mass compared to those taking a placebo. HMB users also shed twice as much fat as nonusers. HMB doesn't only work for strength athletes; it offers benefits to endurance athletes as well. Studies of cyclists and runners show that HMB helped them increase aerobic performance and reduced the telltale signs of muscle damage that are associated with prolonged and strenuous activity. Scientists are not sure how HMB works. Some suspect that it helps prevent *proteolysis,* a natural process that breaks down muscle cells after an intense workout, which quickly erodes all your hard work. A recent study suggests that HMB may be involved in the production of intracellular cholesterol within the muscle, which may explain how it accelerates muscle repair. Here's why: Although too much cholesterol can be harmful, cholesterol is essential for the repair of *cell membranes,* the protective covering of all cells, including muscle cells. HMB may stimulate the production of cholesterol in muscle cells just when it needs it the most—to repair overworked cells.

HMB is not just for people who are already in great shape, it may be just the edge older exercisers need to get sleeker and stronger. From age thirty, adults lose an average of 6 percent muscle mass per decade. That's why we tend to look flabby! Resistance training is a great way to maintain muscle mass, but it does get harder as you get older. The good news is, HMB may be a useful tool in helping older adults hold onto their muscle, as long as they also exercise. Two recent studies have examined the effects of HMB on men and women over seventy. In one study, thirty-one men and women seventy and over participated in two-day-per-week resistance training for eight weeks. Some were given 3 grams HMB daily, others were given a placebo. After four weeks of training, the HMB increased leg strength over the placebo group. After eight weeks, they had a greater increase in lean muscle mass and a greater decrease in fat than the placebo group. In a second study of older adults, researchers examined whether resistance training could improve the ability of older people to perform real-life tasks, such as getting up from a chair—appropriately called the Get up and Go Test. Older adults who participated in a resistance-training program showed a 2 percent improvement in the Get up and Go Test, while those who took HMB showed a 7 percent improvement. So, if you're already taking HMB, tell your parents or grandparents about it!

HMB is not a magic pill—it only works if you work with it. This supplement is for people who are dedicated to pursuing an exercise program. It will enhance your results, but it won't do the job for you.

As far as safety is concerned, HMB wins with flying colors. As of this writing, there have been more than fifteen studies of HMB over the past decade. A recent analysis of nine human studies in which participants consumed 3 grams of HMB daily for three to eight weeks found that HMB did not adversely affect any measure of health, including liver function. In fact, HMB decreased overall cholesterol levels by about 6 percent, and LDL, or bad cholesterol, by 7 percent. The only side effect from HMB was that respondents reported they were in better moods! (As good as HMB is, it has never been tested on pregnant or lactating women, who should not use this or any other supplement without consulting their physicians.)

The buzz is that HMB combined with creatine is even more effective. I'm waiting to see the studies, but the early word is that these two supplements were meant for each other.

HMB may have applications in serious medicine. A study presented at the World AIDS Conference (1998) showed that the combination of HMB, arginine, and glutamine can restore lost muscle mass in AIDS patients confined to bedrest. Currently, HMB is being investigated as a treatment for wasting syndrome in cancer patients.

Possible Benefits

Makes bigger muscles, burns fat.
Increases strength.
May boost mood.
May help prevent disease by lowering bad cholesterol.
Reduces blood pressure.
May help older people retain muscle strength along with exercise.

How to Use It

HMB is a patented product licensed under several private labels. To ensure that you are getting the real thing, the label should carry the Patent Number 5,348,979. Take four 1000 mg. tablets daily.

HOMEOPATHIC GROWTH FACTORS

 Homeopathic growth hormone (also called *signal cell enhancers*)—is the marriage of nineteenth-century and twenty-first century medicine. *Homeopathy* is a system of medicine followed by close to 500 million people worldwide. As I've mentioned, the underlying principle to homoepathy is that like cures like, that is, substances that in large doses can make you sick, in small doses can cure you. Homeopathic remedies are actually very dilute solutions of normally toxic substances that can create the same symptoms that you are trying to cure. Before you dismiss this as hokum, there have actually been several double-blind, clinical studies published in reputable medical journals that confirm the value of homeopathy for some ailments.

As noted Human Growth Hormone* growth hormone treatment offers benefits to older people who are producing less growth hormone, including increased muscle strength, less fat, more energy, and better immune function. The downside is that the side effects of growth-hormone injections can be so unpleasant—not to mention expensive— that it is simply not practical for most people. Recently, one Seattle company developed a form of homeopathic growth hormone (known as *homeopathic signal cell enhancers*) that can be taken orally. Similar to traditional homeopathy, homeopathic growth hormone contains growth factors made by recombinant DNA, but in homoeopathic doses. (A homeopathic dose is quite dilute—a homeopathic preparation that is identified as 10,000X means that it has been diluted tenfold, four times. In homeopathic terms, the more diluted a substance is, the more powerful it becomes.)

So, does homeopathic growth hormone work? Biomed Comm, the Seattle company that developed homeopathic signal cell enhancers recently conducted three studies on their product, published in the December 1999 *Alternative and Complementary Therapy*, a peer-reviewed medical journal. These early studies suggest that oral homeopathic growth hormone can produce real and beneficial changes in the body, without side effects, including changes in body shape and composition and improved mood. As noted in the study, "Homeopathic HGH also improved self-perceived measures related to quality of life significantly, such as weight loss, improved vision, increased libido, improved sleep quality, improved breathing, and improved skin softness. Thus, an oral formulation that was at least 4000 times lower in concentration than an injectable HGH provided some of the same benefits of the injectable HGH without its side effects."

These positive results are based on only three studies, which ran three to six weeks. Also, the effects of homeopathic growth hormone are subtle—people may have felt better and lost a few pounds, but it did not turn flab into muscle overnight. If you are young and your body is pumping lots of growth hormone anyway, I don't think this product will do you much good. If you are older and your production of growth hormone is on the decline, it may help reverse the downward spiral, a least a bit. However, if you're overweight, flabby, and sedentary, taking this or any other pill is not going to transform your body.

My final answer? I think this stuff is interesting. If it's not over-hyped and overmarketed, it may attract the attention of physicians who are openminded about using alternative therapies.

Possible Benefits

May offer the benefits of human growth hormone without the side effects.

How to Use It

Take one tablet three times daily. For best results, take the first tablet between 4 to 8 A.M., the second tablet between 2 to 4 P.M., and the third before bedtime.

HORNY GOAT WEED

Okay, stop laughing, this stuff is serious stuff. Horny goat weed is a revered Chinese medicine, known as *ying-yang-huo*. It has been used in China for centuries to treat male sexual problems and fatigue. Recently marketed in the West, horny goat weed is being touted as the herbal Viagra. How did this herb get its colorful name? The story goes that farmers noticed that, after eating the weed, their goats became more sexually active. Human nature being what it is, they decided to try it themselves.

According to animal studies, horny goat weed can raise testosterone levels, increase sperm production and improve circulation, all of which could theoretically improve sexual function in men. There is plenty of anecdotal material contending that it does. Similar to Viagra, horny goat weed may inhibit an enzyme known as *acetylcholinesterase*, which can interfere with sensory nerves, decreasing sexual desire and the ability to have an erection. In fact, some herbalists feel that horny goat weed is so similar in action to Viagra that, like Viagra, it should not be used by people taking nitroglycerin drugs for heart conditions. I'd like to make a point here—simply because something is natural doesn't mean that it isn't powerful. More than half of all prescription medications are derived from herbs, so do not assume that every herb is safe for everyone. Although it's true that herbs tend to be gentler than prescription drugs and cause fewer side effects, if you have a medical problem, please do not use any over-the-counter drug—herbal or not—without first checking with your physician.

Horny goat weed is often sold in formulas combined with maca, muira purama, and other herbal aphrodisiacs.

Possible Benefits

Boosts sexual desire and performance.
Enhances energy.

How to Use It

Take up to three 1000 mg. capsules or powder dissolved in a beverage daily.

HUMAN-GROWTH HORMONE-RELEASING AGENTS

facts Human-growth hormone is available by prescription in the United States. Growth hormone shots are expensive, and can cost anywhere from nine to twelve thousand dollars a year, too pricey for most people. Nevertheless, I am including growth hormone in the Hot Hundred because there are numerous products sold over the counter that purport to contain growth hormone, or claim to stimulate the body's natural production of growth hormone. Before you spend your money on these products, you need to understand what human growth hormone is and what, if anything, these products can do for you.

Growth hormone is made in the pituitary gland, located under your brain. Children have high levels of growth hormone, for good reason—they're still growing! Growth hormone triggers the onset of sexual maturity in adolescents, increases the size of their muscles, and stimulates their bones to grow. Although it is released steadily throughout the day, peak production occurs at night when we are sleeping (yet another reason why sleep is so important). Vigorous exercise also produces a spike in growth hormone. Our levels of growth hormone decrease with age, dropping at a rate of 14 percent for each decade of adult life. The pituitary gland continues to pulse growth hormone thoughout the day, but the peaks don't get as high. By about age sixty, most people produce very little growth hormone. How growth hormone works is not yet fully understood, but it appears to stimulate the liver to produce another hormone, IGF-1 (insulinlike growth factor), which may be responsible for some of the effects attributed to growth hormone.

What we know about growth hormone is based on studies of growth-hormone-deficient children. Kids who do not produce enough growth hormone do not reach normal height or develop properly. Since the 1960s, growth hormone has been used as a treatment to spur the growth of growth-hormone-deficient children. Growth hormone used to be extracted from the pituitary glands of cadavers, but that practice was banned in 1985, when some adults who had been treated with growth hormone in the 1960s began to develop Creutzfeldt-Jakob disease (Mad Cow disease). Recent breakthroughs in genetic engineering made it possible to grow growth hormone in a test tube from cultures using recombinant DNA, but it is very expensive.

Growth hormone's potential as an age-reversing, muscle-building drug captured the imagination of the scientific community in 1990, with the publication of a study headed by Daniel Rudman, M.D. in the *New England Journal of Medicine*. In the study, twenty-one healthy men, ages sixty-one to eighty-one, with low blood levels of IGF-1 were given either growth-hormone injections three times per week for six weeks or were untreated. At the end of six months, Dr. Rudman reported that the men given growth hormone had an 8.8 increase in lean body mass, a nearly 15 percent decrease in fat tissue, a 7 percent increase in skin thickness and a 1.6 percent increase in lower-spine bone density. Dr. Rudman concluded that the drop in IGF-1 was in part responsible for the increase in fat and loss of muscle associated with aging. The National Institutes on Aging sponsored several clinical studies to see if growth hormone could prevent older people from becoming frail. The results were disappointing, primarily due to the nasty side effects of growth hormone: sore joints, swollen legs and ankles, and carpal-tunnel syndrome. In fact, many participants dropped out of growth-hormone studies because they couldn't tolerate the side effects. Although other researchers have confirmed that growth hormone can improve muscle tone, interestingly, it did not appear to improve strength.

The initial enthusiasm over growth hormone was further dampened when some researchers expressed concern that there could be a link between elevated IGF-1 levels and prostate cancer.

Proponents of growth hormone claim that these studies used doses that were well beyond normal physiological doses, which caused the high rate of side effects. Physicians who use growth hormone in their practice say it needs to be dosed carefully for each individual. These physicians also say that if IGF-1 levels are restored to normal physiological range, there is no increased risk of cancer. So far, studies show that growth hormone is of greatest value to people who are already frail and sick. There are no studies showing that growth hormone can enhance strength or performance in young, healthy people. Nevertheless, some body builders and athletes use it. If you are buff to begin with, growth hormone is not going to do anything for you that other supplements can't as well for a lot less money. Yet, many older people swear by growth-hormone injections—saying they make them look and feel younger.

Several companies have marketed so-called growth-hormone-releasing agents at a fraction of the cost of real growth hormone. These supplements often include amino acids (like arginine, ornithine, and lysine), which have been shown in studies to stimulate the release of growth hormone and/or other *growth factors*, substances that regulate cell activity. Some (but not all) manufacturers of these products will provide studies showing that their product boosts levels of IGF-1, a marker for growth hormone levels. A handful will produce unpublished studies showing that growth-hormone-releasing agents can actually change body composition and enhance weight-loss efforts. They will also offer anecdotal reports from happy users. Do they work? Who knows!

The growth-hormone story may just be beginning. There are several pharmaceutical companies looking to develop growth hormone releasing agents that have scientific backing.

Possible Benefits

May enhance muscle strength.
May reverse some common symptoms of aging.
Helps with weight control

How to Use It

Real growth hormone is administered by injection. Protocols vary from doctor to doctor. Frankly, I don't recommend it. There are many reputed growth-hormone boosters, such as arginine, ornithine, and glutamine. In fact, there are so many products that it is impossible for me to detail each and every dose. Follow the directions given for each.

HYDROXYCITRIC ACID

 Hydroxycitric acid (HCA), which is synthesized from the rind of the garcinia cambrogia, is similar to citric acid found in citrus fruits. Also called *Malabar tamarind, garcina* is a pumpkin-shaped fruit used throughout Asia as a condiment with dishes such as curry. HCA is sold as a single supplement, and is also included in many weight-loss formulas, diet bars, sports drinks, and chewing gum. Preliminary research suggested that HCA inhibits the synthesis of fatty acids by the liver, which should theoretically promote weight loss. HCA was also reputed to be an appetite suppressant—at least it worked that way in animal studies. Early, uncontrolled studies of humans also produced some positive results, and there are lots of anecdotal reports of its effectiveness. The problem is, HCA flunked an important test conducted by Steven B. Heymsfield, Ph.D., at the St. Luke's Roosevelt Hospital Weight Management Center. In the study of 165 overweight patients, reported in the *Journal of the American Medical Association*, sixty-five patients took 1500 mg. HCA, and the rest were put on a placebo. Both groups were on a low-fat, high-fiber diet. The researchers reported that the group taking HCA did not lose more weight than the group taking the placebo. HCA supporters contend that the study was not conducted well. First, they say that the HCA dose was too low. Second, they feel that the high-fiber content of the diet interfered with the proper absorption of HCA. Dr. Heymsfield pointed out that he merely followed the directions on the bottle from the health-food store! Since there haven't been any other studies to date, we don't know if their points are valid.

What's a consumer to do? We're back to what I've been saying all along (not just in this book, but in all my books). When it comes to weight loss, there is no magic bullet. It's a combination of eating the right foods, in the right amount, and expending the right amount of energy.

I haven't given up on HCA. I think it might have a synergistic effect when combined with other fat burners.

Possible Benefits

May enhance weight loss; however, it's still unproven.

How to Use It

Take one 500–750 mg. capsules up to three times daily, one-half hour before meals.

IPRIFLAVONE

For reasons that I can't quite understand, ipriflavone (7-isopropoxy-isoflavone) is being touted as a hot, new, body-building supplement. Ipriflavone is a synthetic compound made from *isoflavones*, phytoestrogens found in soy. It's supposed to boost testosterone levels. The muscle-building claim is based on studies performed by a Hungarian pharmaceutical company, which showed that ipriflavone caused muscle gain in various animals. However, no studies have been done on humans. It's true that soy protein is mildly anabolic (see page 143) but whether it is superior to other forms of protein as a muscle builder has not been proven. At least, there are no convincing studies to date. In reality, any high-protein diet is going to boost free testosterone levels in men. There is no dispute, however, that ipriflavone is very good at building bone in both men and women.

Of course, this is of great interest to postmenopausal women who are at greatest risk of developing *osteoporosis*, the bone-thinning disease that makes them vulnerable to fractures, but men aren't immune to this bone-breaking disease. Whether you are male or female, you need to worry about osteoporosis. When you are young, old bone is constantly being broken down and new bone is constantly being produced in a process called *remodeling*. By our thirties, we begin to lose bone faster than we can replace it. Although bone loss progresses faster in women than in men, and men start out with more bone to begin with, they also lose significant amounts of bone in their later decades. Just like women, men with thinning bone can break a hip or a vertebrae and end up debilitated. If you take care of yourself, this doesn't have to happen.

Weight-bearing exercise helps to build bone. There is also compelling evidence that ipriflavone can help prevent osteoporosis. So if you don't want to end up a frail, bent-over, little old lady or man, keep reading.

More than one hundred animal and human studies, most performed in Europe, have shown that ipriflavone helps prevent bone loss and in fact, can *increase* bone tissue. It appears to suppress the cells that break down bone. Ipriflavone is particularly effective when combined with *calcium*, a mineral essential for the maintenance and repair of bone. In a major clinical trial, 453 women showing signs of bone loss were given 600 mg. ipriflavone and 1000 mg. calcium daily, or just calcium alone for two years. The women taking calcium alone showed a decrease in bone mass; in other words, they were still losing bone. The women taking ipriflavone and calcium did not experience any more bone loss, which strongly suggests that ipriflavone may prevent osteoporosis.

More good news: Ipriflavone may lower cholesterol and help protect against cancer.

When should you start taking ipriflavone? Women experience the most rapid loss of bone within the first five years following menopause. It makes sense to start taking calcium and ipriflavone as soon as you reach your forties and are close to menopause. As for men, if you have a strong family history of osteoporosis, or have taken steroids (which accelerate bone loss) consider taking extra calcium and ostiflavone once you hit your fifties.

Ipriflavone is often sold under the name Ostivone. There are several brands to choose from. It makes sense to buy a combination formula that includes 1000 mg. calcium and 400 IU vitamin D.

Possible Benefits

Halts bone loss.
May stimulate new bone formation.

How to Use It

Take three 300 mg. daily.

IRON

Women and marathon runners, pay attention! You are at risk of developing iron-deficiency anemia. If you are a vegetarian, the odds of being iron deficient are even greater. Iron is an essential nutrient for everyone, but it is of special importance to athletes. Iron transports oxygen to muscle cells, where it is used to make energy. Without iron, you can't make ATP, the fuel that runs the body. Iron deficiency could result in anemia, which will leave you feeling tired, run down, and are more susceptible to infection. Obviously, it's going to interfere with your physical and mental performance. Teenage girls and women who work out hard are prone to develop iron-deficiency anemia because they lose additional iron through menstruation. For reasons that are not fully understood, male marathon runners are also at greater risk of developing iron-deficiency anemia than other athletes.

One obvious solution is to be sure that you get enough iron-rich foods in your diet. Iron is found in foods such as red meat, pork, oysters, beans, iron-fortified grains, green leafy vegetables, dried fruit, and, of course, liver. *Heme iron*, the kind found in animal products, is more easily absorbed than iron found in plant foods, which is why vegetarians may not get enough iron. Vitamin C will help improve the absorption of iron. Calcium and caffeine can interfere with the absorption of iron.

If you suspect that you are deficient in iron, check with your doctor. First, the primary symptom of iron deficiency, fatigue, could be a symptom of another problem. Second, consuming too much iron can be dangerous. In fact, it can increase the risk of heart disease (especially in men) and colon cancer. So, take iron only when you really need it.

Possible Benefits

Iron is needed for energy.

How to Use It

The Daily Value (DV) for iron is 10 mg. daily for men; 15 mg. daily for women eleven to fifty; 10 mg. for postmenopausal women, and

30 mg. for pregnant women. If you are diagnosed with iron-deficient anemia, your doctor will prescribe an iron supplement.

· ·

7-KETO

· ·

7-keto is a chemical analog of DHEA, the most abundant steroid hormone in the body, produced by the adrenal glands, skin, and brain (page 66). 7-keto, the result of decades of research by scientists at the University of Wisconsin, is being promoted as a muscle-building, fat-burning, brain-boosting, energizing supplement. If you cut through the hype, however, there is some interesting science behind 7-keto.

Real DHEA breaks down into two other hormones: estrogen and testosterone. Both estrogen and testosterone can stimulate the growth of hormone-sensitive cancers, which makes DHEA a bad choice for people at high risk of developing certain types of cancer. In some cases, DHEA can produce too much estrogen in men and too much testosterone in women, which can produce undesirable side effects. 7-keto, however, does not convert into steroid hormones in the body; in fact, it is not a hormone at all.

Will 7-keto help you lose weight and retain lean muscle tissue? Animal studies have yielded positive results, but there have been few human studies. One small study conducted at Greenwich Hospital in Connecticut, studied the effect of 7-keto on thirty overweight adults. In the eight-week studies, fifteen people were given 200 mg. 7-keto daily and fifteen were given a placebo. Both groups exercised for one hour, three times per week. At the end of the study, the group taking 7-keto lost significantly more body weight and fat than the placebo group. Interesting, the 7-keto group had higher levels of T3, the active form of thyroid hormone, which suggests an increase in metabolism. Before we can say that 7-keto is a *bona fide* thermogenic agent, there must be a few more controlled studies involving more people! The manufacturers tell us that they are in the works.

7-keto may also help retain muscle mass in a different way—it appears to control *cortisol*, the stress hormone that hurls the body into a catabolic state. The combination of stress and cortisol makes people hungrier, and forces the body to burn lean tissue, causing muscle wasting. At the same time, it makes you hold onto fat! The cortisol response made sense back in the days when cavemen roamed the veldt with wild animals and didn't know when or where their next meal was coming from. It was eat or be eaten! Today, our body's response to cortisol is very destructive in a society in which food is abundant, stress is a way of life, and junk food is everywhere. Several studies confirm that 7-keto can reduce elevated cortisol levels, which theoretically should help maintain muscle.

The most documented benefit of 7-keto is its positive effect on immune function. 7-keto boosts levels of key immune cells that are critical for fighting disease and maintaining health. It is well known that endurance athletes—particularly marathon runners—run the risk of getting respiratory infections after weeks of intense training. They are literally *run down*. I feel that 7-keto could be a useful tool in helping to maintain a strong immune system.

As far as its brain-boosting claims, animal studies document that 7-keto can improve memory. Recent studies confirm that mice given 7-keto learned tasks faster and were better able to negotiate their way out of maze than those taking a placebo.

Possible Benefits

May enhance fat burning, weight loss.
Controls stress.
Boosts immune function.
Improves memory.

How to Use It

Even though 7-keto is not a hormone, some integrative physicians recommend that you have your natural DHEA levels checked before taking 7-keto. If your levels are normal, there is no need to take more. Many people over forty will find that they have lower than normal levels of DHEA, in which case, 7-keto may help fill the void.
The usual dose is 25 to 50 mg. daily.

LEUCINE

 If you read the label of your protein-powder supplement, you will likely see leucine listed in the ingredients. *Leucine* is an essential amino acid, which means that since your body cannot manufacture it on its own, you must get it from food. Leucine is especially important for people who want to build muscle and maintain lean tissue. This amino acid inhibits the breakdown of muscle proteins that often occur after injury, severe stress, or illness. Many athletes believe that it can speed their recovery after an intense workout. Although there is no evidence that leucine will make you bigger, it will certainly help prevent the breakdown of muscle after rigorous exercise. Leucine is not only important for the very fit, but can be a lifesaver to people who are recovering from trauma or surgery. When fasting, the body can use leucine instead of glucose as an energy source. Leucine is essential for a healthy liver; low levels of this amino acid are found in people with liver disease.

Interestingly, leucine is also present in opiatelike chemicals in the brain, called *enkephalins*, which help boost mood and block pain. All protein-rich foods are a good source of leucine.

You can take leucine by itself, or in a protein powder, or a formula containing other branched-chain amino acids.

Possible Benefits

Helps maintain muscle.
Speeds recovery from workout.

How to Use It

Take 500–3000 mg. daily, between meals.

LIPOIC ACID

facts It's called the *energizing antioxidant*. Everyone should take *lipoic acid* (alpha lipoic acid) as part of a daily supplement regimen, but if you work out on a regular basis, you need it even more. Lipoic acid is instrumental in the production of energy by the cells of the body. It helps break down sugar for the production of *ATP*, the fuel that runs the body. In fact, without lipoic acid, cells cannot utilize energy and will shut down. After vigorous exercise, cells need extra energy for repair and recovery. If you don't have enough ATP, you cannot build new muscle. If you don't have enough lipoic acid, you will not have enough ATP.

Athletes and body builders also need lipoic acid for its antioxidant activity. The harder you work out, the more oxygen you burn. The more oxygen you burn, the more free radicals you produce. If left unchecked, free radicals can destroy healthy tissue, including muscle. If you don't have enough antioxidants to mop up the free radicals, over time, all your hard work may be for nothing!

Lipoic acid also enhances the effect of other key antioxidants, vitamin C and E. In addition, it is one of the few substances that can significantly boost levels of *glutathione*, essential for both a healthy immune system and muscle growth.

Lipoic acid's most important job in the body may be to protect us against the damaging effects of *glucose*, a sugar our body produces from food. We can't live without glucose anymore than we can live without oxygen, but glucose comes with a high price tag. When proteins are exposed to glucose, they trigger a chemical reaction that causes the cross linking of proteins, called *advanced glycation end products* (AGEs). AGEs can damage healthy organs, and even cause age spots! AGEs occur everywhere—the eyes, arteries, muscles, and brain. To compound the problems, AGEs also promote the formation of free radicals, which cause even more destruction. Fortunately, there is a weapon against AGEs—lipoic acid. Lipoic acid helps control excess glucose by improving the utilization of glucose by muscle cells. Studies show that it can also reduce AGEs damage in animals and humans.

Lipoic acid is naturally produced in the body, but production falls off as we age. It is found in small amounts in potatoes, spinach, and red meat, but you can't get enough from food alone. Take lipoic acid supplements, or take an antioxidant formula that includes lipoic acid.

Possible Benefits

Essential for the body to produce energy.
Great antioxidant.
Helps control damaging effect of glucose.

How to Use It

Take two 50 mg. tablets daily. I take a multiple antioxidant supplement with 50 mg. alpha lipoic acid.

MACA

 Dubbed the *Peruvian ginseng* (although it is unrelated to the ginseng family), maca is a cruciferous plant native to Peru. It is a member of the same plant family that includes broccoli, cauliflower, cabbage, and brussels sprouts, but for those of you who go "yuck" at the mere mention of these vegetables, I promise that you won't ever have to eat the stuff. (Once I tell you what maca does, though, many of you will willingly gobble it up!) Maca is a sexual enhancer that works well for both men and women. For more than two thousand years, the Incas have known about the power of maca, and shared this information with the Spanish conquistadores. Recently, maca has been discovered by modern scientists.

The maca plant is grown in the central highlands of Peru, known for its high altitude, thin air, and difficult climate. However, people and animals who live there do not suffer from some of the usual ailments associated with high altitude, notably infertility and a high rate of miscarriage. Why? For centuries, the good health of these Peruvians was attributed to their maca-rich diet. Fresh maca root can be baked or roasted, or dried and boiled in milk to make a porridge or in hot water to make a beverage. What's so special about maca? Maca is a great source of amino acids, and minerals like iron, magnesium, and calcium. It also contains sterols, the building blocks of hormones; and chemicals called *aromatic isothiocyanates*, which may be natural aphrodisiacs. For centuries, maca has been touted as a panacea that could boost energy, restore sexual function, and help relieve rheumatoid arthritis and memory problems. Researchers suspect that it helps normalize hormone levels in both sexes. In fact, Peruvian doctors prescribe maca to women suffering from perimenopausal and menopausal symptoms. Interestingly, the same herb used to treat so-called female complaints is also being embraced by athletes and bodybuilders looking for greater stamina!

Maca is one of the few herbal aphrodisiacs that have been subjected to scientific testing that passed with flying colors. In the 1960s, Peruvian researchers documented that maca increased fertility rates in animals. An April 2000 study published in *Urology*, a respected, peer-reviewed journal reported that rats treated with a maca extract (produced by MacaPure™) showed significant improvement in erectile dysfunction, as well as increased libido. Rats given maca in their chow had more frequent and rapid erections than rats fed a normal diet. Remarkably, the maca rats performed better than rats given testosterone!

Of course, maca has not been tested on humans but, given the fact that it has been used for thousands of years safely, with no known toxic effects, there's no reason not to try it and see if it works for you. I know a lot of people who swear by this stuff! What I like about maca is that it doesn't have any of the potential negative side effects of Viagra.

Possible Benefits

Natural aphrodisiac.
May help erectile dysfunction.
Improves mental and physical endurance.
Great for midlife women.

How to Use It

Take up to three 525 mg. capsules daily.

MAGNESIUM

facts Is magnesium the mineral for a better workout and more energy? *Magnesium* is essential for converting blood sugar into energy, effective nerve and muscle functioning, manufacturing proteins, and building bone. Magnesium is especially important for maintaining normal blood pressure and a healthy heart. Recent studies suggest this mineral may help enhance athletic performance.

In a recent study, twenty-six untrained men were either given magnesium supplements or a placebo. The strength of the men was assessed prior to beginning strength training. At the end of a seven-week training period, although both groups of men showed improvement in strength, those that took the magnesium showed significantly greater improvement, not just in strength, but in lean body mass. In other words, they had more muscle.

A study of competitive rowers found that magnesium supplements enhanced their performance and increased their stamina. More studies are needed to determine whether magnesium is a true ergonomic aid but, since it is good for you in so many other ways, it makes sense to add it to your daily supplement regimen. Magnesium is not safe for everyone. Do not use magnesium if you have kidney problems. Also, stick to my recommended dose; excess magnesium can cause severe diarrhea, particularly in people prone to stomach problems.

Athletes that are trying to reach a specific weight often use diuretics or water pills, which can wash essential minerals out of the body. I do not recommend that anyone do this—it can alter the natural mineral balance in your body, which can be life threatening. Many people with high blood pressure, however, take prescription diuretics to lower their blood pressure. If you do use water pills, prescription or otherwise, talk to your doctor about taking a mineral supplement, including magnesium, to replenish the lost minerals.

Do you get a lot of muscle cramps? Magnesium can help prevent muscle cramps, or lessen their severity.

Good food sources of magnesium include green, leafy vegetables; curry powder; bananas; grains; nuts; and seafood. The DV (Daily

Value) for magnesium for adult men is 350 mg., 400 mg. for teenage boys between the ages of fifteen and nineteen. The DV for women is 280 mg. and 300 for teenage girls between the ages of fifteen and nineteen. Due to the poor modern diet, many people do not get the DV for magnesium.

Possible Benefits

Improves athletic performance.
Helps build muscle.
Great for your heart.

How to Use It

Take one 400 mg. tablet or capsule daily.

METHIONINE

 Methionine (also called L-methionine) is an essential amino acid that you may see listed on the ingredient label of protein supplements. There's no shortage of methionine in the food supply—it's abundant in meat, fish, and dairy products. Methionine is particularly important to body builders and athletes because it is essential for the production of *creatine*, the protein that is necessary for energy production and muscle building (page 62). Methionine may also boost levels of glutathione, the antioxidant that is depleted during times of intense physical activity. It's also important for liver and kidney function.

Methionine is also the building block of SAM-e, the natural antidepressant and antiarthritic supplement that is growing in popularity (page 139). When taken with three B vitamins (folic acid, B6, and B12), methionine can help control levels of *homocysteine*, an amino acid which can increase the risk of heart disease, cancer, and Alzheimer's disease.

Possible Benefits

Boosts levels of creatine.
Important for a healthy liver.

How to Use It

Take 500 mg. daily, one hour before or one hour after eating.

· ·
MSM
· ·

facts — Participating in a sport and performing regular exercise, like strength training, power walking, or running is a terrific way to keep your muscles strong, your body sleek, and your mind sharp. As I noted, however, there's a downside to exercise. The harder you work your body, the greater the likelihood of injury. I'm not just talking about the usual strains, sprain, and bone fractures but that, if you constantly beat up your joints, you're increasing the risk of developing osteoarthritis. The knee pain or injury you suffer at age forty or fifty often dates back to years of misuse and abuse of your body!

Methylsulfonylmethane (MSM) is a supplement that can help protect against the negative side effects of exercise. MSM is a naturally occurring sulfur that is ubiquitous in nature and also one of the most abundant elements in the human body. Although it is found in many foods, including milk, coffee, tea, chocolate, and green vegetables, it is often destroyed by cooking. For thousands of years, sulfur has been used as a healing agent. Today, people still soak in sulfur-rich mineral hot springs to relieve arthritis and sore, aching muscles.

The sulfur in MSM is critical for building healthy cells; forming collagen and other body tissues; and producing enzymes, vitamins, and amino acids; the building blocks of protein. Recent studies suggest that, when taken in higher amounts as a supplement, MSM is a natural pain reliever that reduces inflammation and promotes healing

A preliminary study conducted by Dr. Ronald M. Lawrence, M.D., Ph.D., author of *The MSM Miracle*, showed that MSM may speed the recovery of athletic injuries. In the double-blind, placebo-controlled study of twenty-four injured patients, half were given MSM daily and the other half a placebo. Neither doctors nor patients knew which patients were taking MSM, and which were not. Both groups were treated with similar therapy, including chiropractic manipulation, ultrasound, and muscle stimulation at each doctor's visit. Of the twelve patients who took the placebo, only four graded their symptom reduction as excellent or good. Of the twelve patients who took MSM, seven graded their symptom reduction as excellent or good. What's even more telling is the fact that the patients taking MSM required fewer visits to the doctor—3.25 visits on average, compared with 5.25 visits for the placebo takers.

MSM can also help speed recovery after a vigorous workout. A recent study found that recovery time in marathon runners given MSM dropped by 75 percent! Although MSM can't eliminate post-workout pain, it can significantly reduce pain from overworked, sore joints and muscles.

MSM not only helps relieve short-term injuries, but has also proven to be a powerful treatment for osteoarthritis. In a study of twelve osteoarthritis patients, Dr. Stanley W. Jacob, Gerlinger Professor in the Department of Surgery at Oregon Health Sciences University, a leading MSM researcher, reported that patients taking MSM experienced a comparable level of pain relief as those taking 2400 mg. Motrin, but without the side effects, which include stomach upset and ulcers.

There is also promising evidence that MSM may help prevent osteoarthritis in the first place. Mice fed a 3 percent solution of MSM in their drinking water from ages two to five months showed no degeneration of the articular cartilage, as compared to 50 percent among a control group drinking untreated water. If MSM works this way in humans, it could help promote the regeneration of cartilage, thereby both relieving the symptoms of arthritis, while healing the joint.

Possible Benefits

Reduces pain from arthritis and sports injuries.
Speeds healing of sprain and strains.
Reduces inflammation.
Promotes regrowth of articular cartilage.
Speeds up recovery after a workout.

How to Use It

Take one to three 1000 mg. tablets daily. I take a formula that contains vitamin C complex, to ensure efficient absorption.

NAC

 If you're an endurance athlete who is constantly getting respiratory infections, *n-acetyl-cysteine* (NAC) may be your best friend. NAC is an acetylized form of the amino acid cysteine. NAC may be new to the supplement shelves, but it's not new medicine. It has been used in hospitals for more than two decades as a treatment for cystic fibrosis and acetaminophen poisoning. (Although acetaminophen is safe for most people, at very high doses it can poison the liver by depleting it of *glutathione*, an important antioxidant critical for ridding the body of toxins.) NAC is a terrific way to boost glutathione levels, thereby saving the liver.

Glutathione is also important for maintaining a strong immune system. In fact, after a very strenuous workout, glutathione levels often drop in endurance athletes, particularly if they have been overtraining for a race or other event. It's no coincidence that endurance athletes are also prone to respiratory infections after the competition—the depletion in glutathione leaves them vulnerable to every germ that comes their way. Taking NAC supplements from training sessions through competition can help restore glutathione, thereby protecting against colds and other infections. NAC is great at breaking up congestion in the nose and chest. It thins out mucus, providing great relief for head colds and respiratory ailments.

The fact that NAC can keep you healthy is a good enough reason to include it in the Hot Hundred, but some studies suggest that it may do much more. In fact, it may help increase endurance and build muscle. Studies show that NAC can reduce the exercise-induced increase in free radical production that are a by-product of increased oxygen use. The more you exercise, the more oxygen you burn, and the more free radicals float around your body. Free radicals can promote muscle fatigue and interfere with recovery. NAC, which boosts glutathione, can help prevent the negative effects of exercise, enabling you to get the full benefit of your workout.

NAC is also good for your heart. It lowers levels of *homocysteine*, an amino acid linked to heart disease, stroke, and cancer. It also helps reduce high cholesterol levels.

Possible Benefits

Restores glutathione after an intense workout.

Prevents respiratory infections.

Speeds recovery from colds and flu.

How to Use It

Take two 500 mg. capsules daily during periods of physical stress. If you are sick, take four 500 mg. capsules daily.

NADH

facts

Is your energy gauge running low? This peak perform-ance supplement may prove to be just what the doctor or-dered! *Nicotinamide adenine dinucleotide* (NADH) is a patented form of the most active form of vitamin B3. NADH is a co-en-zyme that stimulates energy production by restoring cellular stores of ATP, the fuel that runs the body. *Enzymes* are proteins that bring about chemical changes; a *co-enzyme* works with enzymes to speed things up.

NADH is found in all living cells, and is abundant in such foods as meat, fish, and poultry. B vitamins are notoriously fragile and are often destroyed by cooking, which is why they need to be taken in the form of supplements.

In a recent study, NADH supplements were tested on women with chronic fatigue syndrome (CFS), a condition characterized by debili-tating fatigue of no known medical origin, lasting more than six months. Symptoms include muscle weakness, muscle pain, and an in-ability to concentrate. Although many doctors suspect that CFS may be triggered by extreme stress or a virus, the cause of this ailment is still a mystery. Why try NADH on patients with CFS? Some researchers be-lieve that CFS is due to the inability of the body to produce enough ATP. In a study conducted at Georgetown University School of Medi-cine, researchers gave twenty-six patients 10 mg. of NADH (in the form Enada, a patented brand) once daily for four weeks. After a four-week break from NADH, the patients were given a placebo. Out of the twenty-six participants, eight felt much better while taking the NADH as compared to two who felt better on the placebo. The one thing that NADH did not improve was muscle strength. The question that remains is whether NADH can increase energy production in healthy people. Although there have not been any serious studies to date, there is anecdotal evidence that it can enhance stamina in some people. Since NADH is also an antioxidant (good for you anyway) and is completely nontoxic taken at prescribed dosages, try it for a month and see if it has the same effect on you.

NADH may not produce bigger muscles, but it may improve your brain power. It boosts production of *neurotransmitters*, important brain chemicals involved in learning, alertness and concentration. People who take NADH claim that it makes them feel more focused, and improves memory and recall. In fact, NADH is being tested on patients with Alzheimer's disease and Parkinson's disease to see if it can prevent further degenerative changes.

Some studies suggest that NADH can protect against liver damage from excessive alcohol consumption. In particular, NADH is supposed to protect against alcohol's negative effect on testosterone production—too much alcohol can block production of testosterone, which can lead to excess body weight and flabby muscles. (Frankly, I wouldn't count on anything saving an alcohol-drenched liver. If you drink, do so sparingly and wisely.)

Possible Benefits

Enhances energy.
Improves mental acuity.
Good for liver health.

How to Use It

Take 2.5–5 mg. daily.

OKG

Ornithine alpha ketoglutarate (OKG) is a combination of the amino acid ornithine and alpha ketaglutate, both of which are involved in the production of glutamine and arginine. Some studies suggest that OKG may have a mild anabolic effect by boosting the levels of muscle-building hormones, including growth hormone and insulinlike growth factors. OKG also prevents the breakdown of muscle and enhances immune function. In particular, it increases the activity of key immune cells—macrophages and immunoglobulins. *Macrophages* are large cells residing in organs that, literally, devour foreign invaders. Immunoglobulins glob onto foreign invaders, marking them for destruction by other immune cells. You need them to keep your immune system working well! Do you need OKG for bigger muscles? My hunch is that this supplement may be of greater benefit to people who are ill and are suffering from muscle wasting than those who are healthy and looking to enhance strength.

Amino acids, in general, are important for the maintenance, repair, and growth of muscle. Amino acids are present in foods rich in protein, such as meat, poultry, fish, and beans. Protein-powder supplements are also an excellent source of amino acids.

Possible Benefits

May increase hormones that trigger muscle growth.
Immune booster.

How to Use It

Take 3–5 grams daily.

ORNITHINE

Several peak performance supplements are *amino acids*, the building blocks of protein. There's a reason why protein is so important for athletes and body builders. You can't make muscle without it. If you don't have enough protein, your body will begin to break down the protein you have. No matter how hard you work, you'll have nothing to show for it! *Ornithine* is a *nonessential amino acid*, which means that, theoretically, your body produces enough of it that you do not have to get it from food or supplements. Ornithine's claim to fame is that, when combined with another amino acid, arginine, it can temporarily boost growth-hormone levels.

The question is, does this short spike of growth hormone have any effect on muscle growth? Maybe. In one controlled trial, weight lifters took either 500 mg. ornithine and 500 mg. arginine twice daily, or a placebo. Within five weeks, those taking the ornithine/arginine had a greater decrease in body fat than the placebo takers. The less fat, the more lean muscle. However, the effect is relatively small. (For more information on ornithine, see OKG.) Similar to other amino acids, ornithine also promotes wound healing.

There is no reason to take ornithine by itself but, if you read ingredient labels, you will see that ornithine is included in combination formulas designed for body builders. Now you know what it is!

Possible Benefits

May boost production of growth hormone.

How to Use It

Take 500–1000 mg. between meals or at bedtime.

PANTHOTHENIC ACID

Panthothenic acid, or vitamin B 5, is one of the B-complex vitamins of particular importance for athletes. Panthothenic acid, in conjunction with co-enzyme A, helps convert nutrients into energy. Some studies suggest that a shortage of B vitamins can interfere with performance and stamina, and that active people may need a bit more of the B vitamins than do sedentary folks. Although panthothenic acid is promoted by some manufacturers as an ergonomic aid, no study to date has linked supplemental use with improved athletic performance.

Panthothenic acid is also needed to make the neurotransmitter *acetylcholine*, involved in memory and mood.

Panthothenic acid is abundant in liver, yeast, and salmon, but is also present in smaller amounts in dairy, eggs, grains, and meat. Proponents of the so-called caveman diet contend that our ancestors got a lot more panthothenic acid in their food than is present in the modern food supply and, therefore, everyone needs to take a small amount of supplemental panthothenic acid daily.

Panthethine, a metabolite of panthothenic acid, can lower elevated cholesterol and triglyceride levels, which increase the risk of heart disease. When used as a cholesterol lowering agent, panthethine is taken at high doses under a physician's supervision.

Possible Benefits

Essential for the production of energy by the body.
Too little may interfere with physical performance.

How to Use It

Take a multivitamin with 25–50 mg. panthothenic acid, as well as other B-complex vitamins.

PHEROMONES

 They don't grow muscle, burn fat, tone you up or make you stronger. What they may do is make you more attractive to the opposite sex, but isn't that enough? *Pheromones* are substances excreted by animals (including humans) that affect reproductive behavior. You can't see them or even consciously smell them as you would other odors and scents, yet scientists have proven they exist. We sense them through a little-known organ known as the *vomeronasal organ* (VNO) located in our nasal cavity. Scientists suspected the existence of pheromones as far back as the 1870s, but it wasn't until 1959, that the first animal pheromone was isolated from male moths. Scientists speculated that moths and other animals used pheromones as a form of nonverbal communication, alerting prospective mates that they were ready and willing. In 1986, research biologist Winnifred Cutler, director of the Athena Institute for Women's Wellness in Chester Springs, Pennsylvania, discovered and isolated human pheromones. In fact, Dr. Cutler discovered a way to create a synthetic version of pheromones that appears to be as good as the real thing. The role of pheromones in humans is somewhat more complicated, and not yet fully understood. For instance, research conducted by Dr. Cutler and other scientists have shown that male pheromones are involved in promoting female fertility and regulating menstrual cycles, yet no one is sure precisely how this works. What's even more interesting is the fact that wearing pheromones seem to enhance your appeal to the opposite sex.

In one study published in *Archives of Sexual Behavior*, Dr. Cutler tested the effect of her synthetic male hormones on the sex lives of thirty-eight heterosexual men, ages twenty-six to forty-two. Some were married, some were in ongoing relationships, and some weren't dating, but wanted to be. In the study, seventeen men were given pheromones to add to their aftershave, and twenty-one men were given a placebo to add to their aftershave. Each week for six weeks, the men were asked to report any change in their "experiences with women." After analyzing the results, Dr. Cutler reported that "a significantly higher proportion of pheromone users than placebo users showed an increase over baseline for sexual intercourse and sleeping next to a romantic partner. There was a tendency for a greater number of pheromone users to increase above baseline in petting/affection/kissing and informal dates." In other words, pheromones appear to make you more loveable.

Studies show that pheromones work just as well for women. In another double-blind study, Dr. Cutler found that women who used pheromones topically three times a week reported a significantly higher rate of sexual contact with men than women using a placebo. Dr.Cutler isn't sure whether pheromones make women more receptive to the sexual advances of men, which explains the higher rate of sexual contact, or whether men are more likely to be sexually attracted to women wearing pheromones.

Pheromones aren't just for fun; they are being used by sex therapists to help couples with sexual problems and to give men and women with self-esteem problems a slight edge in the competitive world of dating. Since they're sold over the counter, you can see if they work for you.

Possible Benefits

Make you more attractive to the opposite sex.
Jumpstart your sex life!

How to Use It

Rub a small amount of pheromones on your neck and wrists. A little dab will do you!

· ·

PHOSPHATIDLYSERINE

· ·

facts *Phosphatidlyserine* (PS) is a naturally occurring phospholipid that is an important component of all cell membranes. PS has been dubbed the memory cure, because it can help boost mental function, but recent studies suggest that PS may do much more, especially when it comes to protecting muscle.

By now you know that exercise is a double-edged sword. It's great for your head and your heart. It does trim the fat and help build muscle. Yet, if you exercise too vigorously, too often, it can cause real trouble. When you overtax your body, your adrenal glands respond by pumping more stress hormones. One of those hormones is *cortisol*, which helps provide the energy to fuel your workout, yet does so at a very high price. Cortisol depletes the amount of protein in tissues, stimulating protein breakdown for glucose synthesis. And where is that protein coming from? Your muscles! A little cortisol is helpful—you need the energy boost to make it through physically or mentally stressful times. Excess cortisol, however, can cause the dreaded C word—*catabolism*—which means that your body is literally feeding upon itself. When you're in a catabolic state, you can't maintain, let alone build, muscle.

PS supplementation may help protect against cortisol damage, according to two recent studies. In one study conducted at the University of Naples, Italy, researchers first measured cortisol output in eight healthy young men before, during, and after exercise on a bicycle ergometer. In the second part of the experiment, they gave the men intravenous injections of either PS or a placebo before their workout. While the men were taking PS, they had a significantly lower increase in cortisol production than when they were given the placebo.

In another double-blind, crossover study, ten trained weight lifters were given 800 mg. PS daily for two weeks before a vigorous workout designed to simulate overtraining. After a wash-out period to rid the body of the supplementary PS, the athletes repeated the program, this time taking a placebo instead of PS. Blood samples taken after a work-out showed that cortisol levels were 20 percent lower when the men were taking PS than when they were on the placebo. Researchers noted that while the men were taking PS, they also reported feeling better and had less muscle soreness.

PS is not only good for brawn, but also for your brain, where the highest concentration of PS is found. In a study by Thomas Crook III, Ph.D, a leading PS researcher, in association with Vanderbilt University, Stanford University, and a manufacturer of PS, researchers gave 140 subjects ages ranging from fifty to seventy-five, 100 mg. PS three times daily for twelve weeks. Those taking PS showed significant improvement in their ability to recall telephone numbers, names, faces, and to perform memorization tasks. According to Dr. Crook, PS supplementation brought patients back an average of twelve years in terms of mental function. Interestingly, the researchers reported that people with the most severe memory impairment benefitted the most from PS.

Possible Benefits

Helps control the damaging effects of cortisol.
Boosts brain function.

How to Use It

Take 50–100 mg. up to three times daily, or take in a complex of phosphatidyl inositol, ethanolamine, and cephalin twice daily, as I do.

POTASSIUM

Potassium is a mineral that works with sodium and chloride to maintain the proper fluid balance in the body. These three minerals are called *electrolytes* because they carry an electrical charge—potassium and sodium are positive, and chloride is negative. Potassium is also critical for automatic muscle contractions and maintaining normal blood pressure. You lose potassium through sweat and urination so, when you sweat a lot, you run the risk of potassium depletion. In fact, according to one recent study, endurance athletes lose about 435 mg. of potassium per hour. (Not to worry, you can easily replace it by eating one banana, or one baked potato, each of which contain 450 mg. potassium.) Severe potassium loss can lead to cardiac arrest and death, but that is rare, and usually happens only in cases of long-term fasting or starvation. Mild potassium deficiency may result in fatigue, which could interfere with your ability to perform at your peak. If you use diuretics to make weight—which I don't recommend—you could also be accelerating your potassium loss. The real risk with diuretics is that you will create an electrolyte imbalance, which can have detrimental effects on your health.

Our ancestors ate a diet much higher in potassium than we do, primarily because food processing destroys this important mineral. For example, fresh seafood is rich in potassium and lower in sodium, but canned seafood contains much more sodium than potassium. The same is true of canned vegetables. The moral is, the best source of nutrients are fresh, unprocessed foods. Sports drinks are a good source of potassium (look for those containing more potassium than sodium) as are fresh fruits and vegetables.

Potassium is also critical for the maintenance of bone; a deficiency in this mineral may promote osteoporosis. A major study conducted by the U.S. Department of Agriculture found that men and women who ate the most potassium-rich foods had the highest bone density.

Possible Benefits

Help maintain normal fluid balance in the body.
Help prevent bone loss.

How to Use It

You need 2000 mg. potassium daily—try to get as much from food as possible. To make up for any shortfalls, take one to three tablets twice up to three times daily. (99 mg. elemental potassium is the highest dose sold without a prescription.)

Caution

Excess potassium is excreted by the kidneys. People with kidney problems should avoid taking potassium supplements or eating a potassium-rich diet.

. . . .

PCO

. . . .

facts   *Proanthocyanidins* (PCOs) are a special variety of flavonoids found in the blue, purple, and green pigments of plants. Blueberries, cranberries, and grapes are rich in PCOs, which are the most potent form of flavonoids and, therefore, the most expensive. They may be well worth the price if you want to stave off the ravages of aging. A recent study conducted at the U.S. Department of Agriculture found that rats fed a few blueberries daily showed far fewer signs of mental and physical aging than those who were not. Another study performed at the University of Urbino in Italy, showed that PCOs derived from pine bark made rats stronger, actually increasing leg strength and muscle mass. Okay, so PCOs are great for rats . . . what about humans? At the Oxygen Society Annual Meeting (November 1998) which attracts the world's leading researchers in antioxidants, scientists reported that PCOs derived from pine bark protected aerobic athletes from free radical damage and improved endurance. The athletes in the study took 200 mg. pine bark PCOs daily. As discussed earlier (see Antioxidants), levels of free radicals rise during exercise which, over time, can slow down recovery and injure muscle cells. PCOs not only neutralize free radicals, but actually increase stamina in direct proportion to the degree of suppression of free radicals.

Here's another reason why athletes should consider taking PCOs: They boost immune function, which can be weakened after a rigorous training period.

Possible Benefits

High-quality antioxidants.

Prevents degenerative damage due to free-radical attack.

How to Use It

Take 15–60 mg. daily.

PYRUVATE

 Pyruvate is one of the most controversial peak performance supplements on the market. Manufacturers are tangled in lawsuits over who owns the patent on this product. Researchers are engaged in a war of words over whether pyruvate is effective and at what doses. At the same time, ads appear in fitness magazines claiming that pyruvate is *the* supplement to burn fat, increase endurance, and gain muscle. It's hard to get to the bottom of the pyruvate story, but I can tell you right now that it is no magic pill. You can't simply take this stuff and find that you have become svelte and strong overnight. However, pyruvate may be of some benefit.

Pyruvate is derived from pyruvic acid and is bonded to a mineral for stability, usually calcium, sodium, or potassium. Made naturally in your body, *pyruvic acid* is a by-product of the energy metabolism of sugar and starch. Studies conducted by pyruvate researcher Ronald T. Stanko, M.D., have found that pyruvate can help overweight people shed pounds. In fact, according to Dr. Stanko's studies, high doses of pyruvate given to obese people on a weight-loss regimen can significantly increase both weight loss and fat loss. Other studies conducted by Dr. Stanko have shown that pyruvate can also increase stamina and endurance. In other studies, conducted in different laboratories, however, pyruvate did not perform as well. In fact, in a study sponsored by EAS, a major supplement company, previously sedentary, obese women were put on an exercise regimen that included walking and resistance training. Some of the women took 5 grams calcium pyruvate daily, others took a placebo. The researchers noted that women taking pyruvate were not able to exercise any better, nor did they show more endurance than the nonusers. The only difference between the two groups was a modest improvement in body composition among the pyruvate users. So, at least among overweight women, if pyruvate has any effect, it appears to be a modest one. Nevertheless, any gain in lean muscle tissue is desirable.

There is contradictory evidence as to whether pyruvate is going to make fit people any fitter. In one short-term study of body builders, pyruvate had no effect on endurance. In another study, however, conducted by Douglas Kalman, M.S.R.D., another well-known pyruvate researcher, pyruvate did produce a significant increase in lean mass. In the study of fifty-three men and women, one group took 6 grams of pyruvate daily, another control group took a placebo, and a third group took nothing. All three groups followed a two thousand calorie per day diet and exercised five times a week. At the end of the study, the group taking pyruvate showed an average 3.4 pound increase in lean mass; the other groups showed little change. From these studies, it appears as if pyruvate can help users lose the fat and gain lean tissue as long as they're doing other things, like eating well and exercising. It won't happen overnight, and the effect may not be dramatic, but every little bit helps.

There's also controversy about the dose of pyruvate needed for results. Some of the earlier studies used very high doses of pyruvate (30–60 grams daily), but more recent studies have used much smaller doses (5–10 grams). The downside is that pyruvate is quite expensive, so you can't gorge on the stuff unless you have unlimited resources. The upside is that it appears to be quite safe. In fact, some studies suggest that it can help enhance heart function. So, if you're looking to get lean, and money is no object, it's certainly worth a try.

Possible Benefits

Burns fat but spares lean tissue.
May increase endurance.

How to Use It

Take six to eight 450 mg. capsules daily with meals. (If you have ulcers, don't take pyruvate on an empty stomach.)

REISHI MUSHROOM

 As the saying goes, there's nothing new under the sun! For more than four thousand years, various species of Asian mushrooms have been used as tonics to increase physical and mental strength and ward off disease. Today, one of the most popular of all Asian delicacies—reishi mushroom—is being touted as an ergonomic tool that can help endurance athletes increase stamina and stay healthy. Known in China as the medicine of kings, reishi is often teamed with ginseng in formulas designed for athletes.

Traditional Asian healers have prescribed reishi for people under extreme physical or emotional stress. In Japan, reishi is a respected treatment for numerous ailments, ranging from allergies to high blood pressure to insomnia. An ancient Chinese herbal dating back to the Ming dynasty noted, "long-term taking of Reishi will build a strong, healthy body and assure a long life."

When it comes to endurance athletes, I think reishi is just what the doctor ordered. It not only helps them to better adapt to their stressful environment, but contains powerful immune-enhancing substances that can prevent the immune slump that often occurs after an intense training period. Reishi is a rich source of *beta glucans*, molecules made up of repeating units of glucose or sugar. When beta glucans bind to immune cells, they trigger a strong immune response, enabling the body to better fight off foreign invaders.

Weight lifters take note: Reishi has also been used successfully to lower high blood pressure. The strain of lifting heavy loads can send blood pressure soaring, at least temporarily, which puts a strain on your heart. Reishi may prove to be a tool that can help weight lifters maintain normal blood pressure. (If you have high blood pressure, please talk to your doctor before starting any weight-lifting or exercise program.)

Reishi has also been studied as a potential treatment for cancer, and can help prevent the clogging of arteries that leads to heart disease. Reishi also contains natural anti-inflammatory compounds, which should help reduce muscle soreness after a strenuous workout.

Possible Benefits

Helps you better cope with physical or emotional stress.
Boosts immune function.

How to Use It

Take one 500 mg. capsule daily, or take a combination athletic formula that includes 500 mg. reishi.

RHODODENDRON CAUCASICUM

facts
This unique species of rhododendron has been used for centuries in folk medicine. In China, where it's known as *man-shan-hung*, it's a traditional remedy for respiratory infections. In the Republic of Georgia in Russia, it's made into a tea that is sipped before meals. The Republic of Georgia is famous for its many residents that live to be one hundred and older. The unusually robust older population has attracted the attention of Russian scientists, who scrutinized the eating habits and lifestyle of its people. Rhododendron tea, which is rich in antioxidants, is believed to be one factor in the longevity of residents of Georgia. (Although *Rhododendron causcasium* is safe and has been used in traditional medicine for hundreds of years, some forms of the rhododendron plant are poisonous. Don't try munching on your rhododendrons at home—they will make you sick.)

Russian scientists learned that this special species of the rhododendron plant is a natural fat blocker—it partially inhibits the action of an enzyme needed for fat absorption. However, unlike prescription fat blockers, it works gently and does not have any unpleasant side effects. Rhododendron doesn't eliminate all fat, just some fat. Remember, you need fat to absorb fat soluble vitamins, to make hormones, and to perform countless other tasks in the body. It's the *excess* fat that you don't need!

Rhododendron is also a powerful antioxidant. In particular, it is a rich source of *polyphenol*, a phytochemical shown to protect against heart disease. Polyphenols prevent the oxidation of LDL or bad cholesterol, a risk factor for heart attacks. Studies show that rhododendron works especially well with arctic root (European ginseng) to burn fat and promote the formation of lean muscle mass. Even if you don't diet or exercise, this herbal combination will improve your muscle-to-fat ratio, but the effects are far more dramatic if you eat carefully and do even a small amount of exercise. In the Republic of Georgia, rhododendron is also used to treat arthritis and gout.

Possible Benefits

Can help keep you slim by blocking the absorption of extra fat.
Good for your heart.
Great antioxidant.

How to Use It

Take one 50 mg. capsule rhododendron extract daily before each meal, up to three daily.

RIBOSE

When you work out hard—whether you run, shoot hoops, pump iron, or spin away the afternoon—you use energy and lots of it. Just the way your car runs on gas, your cells run on *adenosine triphosphate* (ATP) the energy currency of the body. Under normal conditions, your body produces enough ATP to keep things humming along nicely. When you're under extreme physical stress, however, your ATP stores may run low, especially in your muscle cells. If you exercise strenuously three to four times per week, your cells may not have ample time between workouts to replenish your ATP supply enough to meet the increased demand. As a result, you will not only tire more easily during your workout, but will not recover as quickly after your workout. Obviously, you need to refill the fuel tank! That's where ribose comes in. *Ribose* is a simple sugar found in all living cells. It is essential for the production of ATP. Although the body produces ribose on its own, under times of extreme exertion, it may need more ribose to make more ATP.

Ribose was originally used as a treatment for cardiac patients to reenergize sluggish heart cells. Oxygen is also essential for the production of ATP. During times of ischemia, when the heart is deprived of adequate oxygen, levels of ATP in heart cells can plummet, and it can take up to ten days to recover. Researchers have reported that supplemental ribose can help jump start the production of ATP in oxygen deficient hearts, thus giving heart cells the energy they need to heal more rapidly. In fact, numerous studies document its effectiveness as a treatment for heart patients. There is not nearly as much scientific evidence supporting the use of ribose for athletes, but there is some. In one small study conducted at Ball State University, two athletes were given supplemental ribose and two were given placebos. For the first three days, the athletes were given ribose or a placebo (30 grams per day, over three doses). In the second phase, also three days long, the athletes engaged in high-intensity exercise twice per day. In the third phase, the athletes continued taking their supplements or placebo, but did not exercise. The athletes who took that supplemental ribose had increased power output and quicker recovery of *adenonine nucleotides*, the building blocks of ATP, than the placebo takers. In other words, they performed better during their workout and replenished their ATP stores faster after exercise. I repeat, this is a small study, but there are some anecdotal reports from endurance athletes suggesting that ribose does make a difference in both energy levels and recovery. Critics of ribose point out that the dose of ribose used in these studies is significantly higher than that recommended by manufacturers. They question whether ribose is effective in these low doses—there are no studies. In high doses, ribose may be too expensive for most consumers.

Who should use ribose? If you workout intensely several times a week and if, in particular, you feel exhausted between workouts, ribose may turn things around. If you work out only one to two times a week and there is a three-day gap between workouts, your body should have enough time to replenish your ATP stores. If you have a heart condition and are working out (under your doctor's supervision, please!), I would recommend using ribose to see if it helps, especially if you feel as if you're running out of steam during your exercise sessions.

Possible Benefits

Enhances performance during workouts.

Speeds recovery.

May help cardiac patients heal faster.

How to Use It

Ribose is available in capsules, liquid, and powder. It has a slightly sweet taste. Ribose is sold as a single supplement, or in combination with creatine monohydrate. (Some athletes feel that ribose works in synergy with creatine, although this has not been scientifically tested.) The usual recommended dose is three to five grams per day, although that's significantly lower than the 30 grams used in studies. High doses (10 grams daily or more) may cause stomach upset. For best results, divide your dose. Take half an hour before exercise and the second half immediately following exercise. If you want to take it once a day, take it after exercise.

· ·

SAM-e

· ·

S-adenosyl methionine (SAM-e) has been widely used in Europe since the 1980s, but was only recently brought to the United States. It's being touted as a treatment for depression and osteoarthritis. What makes SAM-e a peak performance supplement is that it may be one of the few known substances to actually help *prevent* osteoarthritis. Osteoarthritis, also known as *wear-and-tear* arthritis, is caused by the destruction of the *articular cartilage*, the substance that lines the joints and prevents bones from grinding against each other. As the cartilage gets more worn down, bone becomes exposed and the joint space narrows. Joints begin to feel old and creaky. As noted earlier, osteoarthritis is not just a problem of the old. Degenerative joint changes can begin in your thirties. Young, vigorous people who work their bodies hard may also be beating up their joints, thereby unwittingly promoting premature osteoarthritis.

Numerous studies confirm that SAM-e is a highly effective treatment for mild to moderate arthritis, and works as well as many NSAIDs, but without the side effects. A major clinical trial in Germany involving more than twenty thousand osteoarthritic patients found that SAM-e consistently produced excellent results. (Although NSAIDs also control pain and swelling, if used long term, they may actually worsen osteoarthritis by causing more damage to the joint.) Even more compelling is a new German study that suggests that SAM-e may help repair and restore cartilage, the key to controlling osteoarthritis. Fourteen patients with finger osteoarthritis were given 400 mg. SAM-e daily, while seven who were used as a control were not given any medication. After three months, patients were given an MRI to determine the state of their cartilage. Those taking SAM-e showed a small but definite increase in cartilage thickness compared to those not taking any medication.

Does this mean that taking SAM-e early in life can prevent osteoarthritis down the road? We asked this question of Dr. Peter W. Belligmann, M.D., professor at the Institute of Sports Medicine at the University of Landau in Germany and a member of the German Medical Committee for Top Athletes and the German Medical Committee for the Olympic Team. Dr. Belligmann says that no one knows the answer to this question, but that SAM-e may prove to be a useful tool in helping to preserve cartilage. Since SAM-e is very safe, he feels there is no harm in taking it preventively. Dr. Belligmann also feels that it will work well in combination with glucosamine and chondroitin, two other peak performance supplements.

Possible Benefits

Relieves discomfort of osteoarthritis.
May promote formation of new cartilage.

How to Take It

For moderate arthritis pain, take 600 mg. SAM-e daily with meals. Take three 200 mg. tablets three times daily. To prevent osteoarthritis, take 200 mg. SAM-e daily. It can take six to eight weeks to see results.

SELENIUM

 During times of intense exercise, your body uses up its supply of *glutathione*, an important antioxidant critical for both the recovery of muscle and an optimally functioning immune system. *Selenium* is a mineral necessary for the production of the enzyme *glutathione peroxidase*, required to make *glutathione*, the body's primary antioxidant. Without selenium, you can't make glutathione, which is why I am including it as a peak performance supplement. Not that selenium isn't important in its own right! Selenium protects against many different forms of cancer, heart disease, and stroke, so you should be taking this mineral anyway. Recent studies show, however, that selenium is especially important for people who engage in strenuous exercise on a regular basis. In fact, in a study of cyclists who exercised to the point of exhaustion, those who took supplemental selenium showed far less muscle damage than those who did not. Why would selenium protect muscle? By boosting levels of glutathione, selenium protects against the free-radical damage that normally occurs after intense exercise. The same free radicals that slow down muscle recovery, and promote fatigue, can also dampen immune function. Therefore, by taking selenium, you are also giving your overworked immune system a much needed boost.

Selenium also works in synergy with vitamin E, giving you more antioxidant bang for your buck!

Possible Benefits

Boosts levels of glutathione.
Prevents muscle damage.
Enhances immune function.
Prevents heart disease and cancer.

How to Use It

Take 200 mcg. selenium daily.

SODIUM

Sodium is an important mineral in the blood that, along with potassium, helps the body to maintain a normal fluid balance. Table salt is our main dietary source of sodium and, believe me, most of us are not deficient in this mineral. In fact, we consume way too much salt! In some people, a salty diet can increase the risk of high blood pressure. The American Heart Association recommends that you eat no more than 2400 mg. salt per day but, in reality, most Americans eat two to three times that amount without even realizing it. Even if you don't use the salt shaker, there's lots of hidden salt in our modern, heavily processed diet. One meal at a fast-food restaurant can weigh in at 2000 mg. salt! Yet, despite the fact that most of us consume more salt than we need, there are times we may need to consume even more.

The sodium in salt helps cells retain water. This is bad for people who tend to become bloated, but it's great if you're an endurance athlete competing outdoors for long hours in hot weather. When you're hot and sweaty, you lose fluid, as well as important minerals like potassium and sodium. In fact, a marathon runner can lose ten pounds of water weight in one race! Sodium can help prevent dehydration by holding onto water. If you're a marathon runner, you know that organized events have aid stations throughout the run providing water and salty snacks. Sodium and potassium are also included in most sports drinks. If you're exerting yourself for hours in the heat, you run the risk of *hyponatremia*, dangerously low sodium levels, which can lead to dehydration and heat stroke. During the competition, be sure to fortify yourself with the appropriate fluid-replacement beverages.

Possible Benefits

Prevents dehydration.

How to Use It

For best results, look for sports drinks and snacks containing sodium. When you're not sweating up a storm, you do not need extra sodium.

SOY PROTEIN

Okay, I know that some of you may be thinking, "What's soy protein doing in this book? I thought soy was just for women with hot flashes, men worried about their prostates and people with high cholesterol." Think again! Soy protein is being touted as a hot, new muscle builder.

Soybean, a legume, is one of the few plant foods to contain the proper balance of the eight essential amino acids. In fact, the U.S. government recognizes soy protein as an alternative equivalent to meat. Unlike meat, it does not contain saturated fat, which has been linked to an increased risk of heart disease. The best part about soy is that it's also good for you in many other ways. Every mouthful of soy contains a feast of beneficial phytochemicals, including *isoflavones,* hormonelike substances that help balance the body's production of hormones and may also help prevent both prostate and breast cancer. In fact, people who eat the highest amounts of soy foods have the lowest rates of these diseases. Isoflavones may also prevent bone loss which can lead to osteoporosis. In addition, soy also contains two other powerful anticancer compounds, phytic acid and protease inhibitors.

Soy may also prove to be the protein of choice for athletes. The May 2000 issue of *Lets Live* (one of my favorite health magazines) reports that studies conducted at Ohio State University investigated soy protein's effect on muscle breakdown in recreational athletes. After performing aerobic exercise, student athletes had their levels checked for two important markers of muscle cell breakdown, creatine kinase and myeloperoxidase. After establishing an initial baseline, the athletes either received 20 grams of soy protein isolate or whey protein twice a day for three weeks, along with their regular diet. The athletes who took the soy protein showed significantly fewer markers for muscle breakdown. It's not surprising that soy should help maintain muscle. Protein is the key to rebuilding muscle; soy is rich in two amino acids key to muscle recovery, arginine and glutamine. Endurance and strength athletes require more protein than the average person. I think it's a lot healthier to get some of that protein in the form of soy, instead of high-fat meat and dairy products.

Soy protein is a proven cholesterol-lowering agent. Even the conservative FDA is convinced that eating soy may help prevent heart disease and allows soy manufacturers to say so on their products.

This doesn't mean that you have to eat tofu unless you want to. Soy protein isolate is available in powdered form that can be mixed into water or juice. Instead of eating high-fat sausage and burgers, I recommend that you try soy Boca Links and Boca Burgers. They taste great, and they're a whole lot better for you than the real thing.

Possible Benefits

Protects against several different types of cancer.
Helps repair muscle after exercise.
Generally good for you.

How to Use It

Drink a soy shake daily. (Mix two scoops of soy protein in water, low-fat soy or rice milk.)

SPORTS BARS

They're called sports bars, energy bars, meal-replacement bars, and diet bars. You can find them in health-food stores, drug stores, general-merchandise stores, supermarkets, candy stores, and even sporting-goods stores. They come in every flavor under the sun, from chocolate to mocha to peanut butter to berry. And they promise to do everything under the sun, too. They're supposed to give you energy, build muscle, speed recovery from an intense workout, and help you lose weight. The question is, are they all that they are cracked up to be? Of course, the answer is no.

Let me shatter some myths about sports bars. No matter how well formulated a sports bar may be, it's not as good as real food. If you eat well—by that, I mean if you stick to high-quality protein, vegetables, fruits, and unprocessed carbohydrates—you don't need sports bars. But I understand that, in the real world, many people can't always eat the right food at the right time. So, we turn to convenience foods. Here's where sports bars can come in handy. They're a great afterschool snack for kids on their way to soccer practice or lacrosse. They're wonderful for body builders who need a quick pick me up after working out, or as quick energy surge for marathon runners training for a race. However, all sports bars are not created equal, some are better than others, and some are just bad. Here's some tips on how to find the right one for you.

There are three basic categories of sports bars—high-protein bars, high-carbohydrate bars, and glorified candy bars. The high protein bars (Atkins Advantage Bar, Carbs Away Engineered Nutrition Food Bar, Protein Bar, and so on) are for people who are carefully watching their intake of carbs. High protein bars usually contain from fifteen to thirty grams of protein, often in the form of soy protein, whey protein, or egg protein. The higher the protein content, the dryer the texture of the bar, which can make them unappetizing, depending on your palate. Some experts feel that high protein is best for strength athletes who need to build muscle bulk and muscle. The high carbohydrate bars (for example, Harvest Bar, Boulder Bar, Cliff Bar) are primarily marketed to endurance athletes who rapidly burn up carb calories. High carb bars may contain from thirty to fifty grams of carbs. Finally, there are other bars that are no better than candy bars. If you read their labels, you'll see that one of first ingredients is some form of sugar—usually fructose. The problem is, although sugar provides a quick energy burst, the sudden spike in blood sugar results in an equally sharp drop, which will leave you tired and hungry. So, if you're looking for sustained energy, these bars are not going to do the job.

Sports bars are fine for very active people who don't have to worry about their weight, but I don't think any of these bars are great for dieters. Frankly, I think that if you need to lose weight, you must learn how to eat real food in realistic portions. Relying on so-called diet bars may work for a while, but you'll get sick of them pretty fast. They're also pretty high calorie for an afternoon snack. (You're better off eating an apple at 90 calories than a sports bar at 200!)

Some sports bars today are laden with other nutrients, such as glutamine, L-carnitine, ginseng, caffeine, and other vitamins and minerals. Personally, I don't think this is the best way to take supplements-food-processing techniques may alter the dose, so you can never be sure of what you're really getting.

If you do use sports bars, read the labels! Make sure that the bar contains the right mix of protein and carbs for you, and that it is low in sugar. These bars often contain dozens of ingredients. If you have a food allergy be especially careful about reviewing ingredients.

Possible Benefits

High-protein bars are a good source of high-quality protein and relatively low fat.
High-carb bars are good for endurance athletes.
Beats eating pure junk.

How to Use Them

Either before or after a workout.

Caution

Dieters beware! Don't fall into the "if it's a diet bar I can eat it along with everything else and not gain weight" syndrome.

SPORTS DRINKS

Sports drinks are by far the best selling of all peak performance supplements. The granddaddy of sports drinks, Gatorade, has become so popular that it's sold in supermarkets and consumed as a regular beverage! Gatorade, a flavored beverage containing a simple sugar (sucrose) and salt was first used by the Gators, the football team of University of Florida in Gainesville, one of the hottest and most humid places in the country. Today, there are scores of sport drinks on the market. Some are sold as ready-to-drink beverages, others are in powders that need to be rehydrated with water. Although they have become more sophisticated, they all basically do the same things, that is, prevent dehydration and speed recovery.

Any form of physical activity—from running to gardening to cycling—is going to result in the loss of water through sweating, breathing, and urination. The harder you work out, the more fluid you lose. As I mentioned, a marathon runner can lose up to ten pounds of water weight in a single race. Even a small loss in body water can result in fatigue and poor mental and physical performance. So, it's very important to replenish fluid as you lose it. When you sweat, you not only lose water, but important minerals like potassium, sodium, and magnesium. These three minerals are called *electrolytes*, because they have an electrical charge and are critical for normal fluid balance in the body. Ideally, when you replenish fluid, you should also restore lost electrolytes. In addition, many companies are adding other ingredients to sports drinks including vitamins and glutamine, a peak performance supplement.

The question is, is there an advantage to drinking sports drinks over plain water? When tested against water or a placebo, some studies have shown that presweetened, mineral-enriched beverages (like Gatorade) can improve stamina and endurance. If they work for you, use them! If you don't think it makes a difference, stick to water. Some people actually find that sports drinks upset their stomach. My advice, once again, drink water. Manufacturers make a big deal about differentiating between fluid-replacement drinks and recovery drinks. In terms of postexercise recovery, however, I don't think that sports drinks make that big a difference. You can get the same effect from drinking a glass of water and eating a banana, a great source of potassium.

Avoid sports drinks that contain caffeine or carbonation, both have a mild diuretic effect, which defeats the purpose of a sports drink.

Possible Benefits

Prevents dehydration.
May improve performance.

How to Use Them

Drink before, during, and after exercise. I take a powder punch after a workout with MSM complex, carbohydrate, vitamin C, and ginseng to prevent leg cramps and muscle soreness, and to restore lost fluids.

SYNEPHRINE

Synephrine is an extract from one of several species of the plant genus *Citrus aurantium* or *Citrus wilsonii*, also known as *immature bitter orange*, *Zhi shi*, or *sour orange*. The unripened fruit of these plants has been used in Chinese medicine for thousands of years to treat respiratory infections and gastrointestinal problems like indigestion. Synephrine is being touted as a milder version of *ephedrine*, a well-known stimulant. Ephedrine turns up metabolism, which may help burn fat but, in some people, can also raise blood pressure and cause heart palpitations and jitters. Synephrine is reputed to have the fat-burning properties of ephedra without the negative side effects. Synephrine is rarely used as a standalone herb, but is most often combined with other metabolic enhancers, including hydroxycitric acid, yohimbe, and chromium. The question is, does it work? Granted, synephrine has a long history of use in Chinese medicine, but not as a treatment for obesity. Serious studies on synephrine are scarce. One study, conducted at Greenwich Hospital, tested a combination of bitter orange extract (975 mg.), caffeine (528 mg.), and St. John's wort (900 mg.) on overweight but healthy people. Twenty-three test subjects were either assigned the herbal combination daily, a placebo, or nothing. They all ate 1800 calories daily and performed strength-training exercises three times per week. At the end of six weeks, those taking the herbal combination lost more body fat, and had lower cholesterol and triglycerides than those taking the placebo or nothing. This study doesn't really assess the validity of synephrine since it is hard to tease out which ingredient in the herbal mixture worked best. It does show, however, that the combination of ingredients seems to have some value.

Frankly, I don't like the way stimulants make me feel. I don't drink any beverages containing caffeine, so I am not crazy about these products. Metabolic enhancers like synephrine may help reduce body fat—especially if you are overweight—but use them carefully. I understand that these products may be useful for others, but I want you to use them carefully. First, check with your doctor to make sure that you don't have a medical condition (either diagnosed or hidden) that could make these products dangerous. For example, if you have high blood pressure, or a pre-existing heart condition, steer clear of these products. If you have a strong family history of heart disease I would also avoid them. Even if you pass your physical with flying colors, I would not use these products for more than four to six weeks at a time. While you are using them, avoid other stimulants, like caffeinated beverages. If you have any negative side effects, discontinue use.

Possible Benefits

Help turn up metabolism to burn fat.

How to Use Them

Take 3–6 mg. standardized extract daily. Look for products containing 1.5 to 3 percent synephrine. Don't take a metabolic stimulant too close to bedtime—it could interfere with sleep.

T-BOOSTERS

T-boosters are a class of performance supplements reputed to raise testosterone levels. Popular T-boosters include androstenedione and the other andros, DHEA and tribulis terrestis. Undoubtedly, within the first few months after this book goes to press, there may be others on the market. T-boosters are touted as a legal way to get the athletic and sexual boost of anabolic steroids without the negative side effects. Since T-boosters were first brought to market in the 1990s, there have been nagging questions about both their safety and efficacy. I will try to answer some of those questions here.

The benefits of T-boosters are directly related to the effects of testosterone, therefore, to fully understand what T-boosters are, you need to know about the real thing. *Testosterone* is a hormone produced by both men and women, although men make much higher quantities. Known as the male sex hormone, testosterone is critical for male sexual development, as well as secondary male sexual characteristics, including body hair and muscle development. Testosterone is essential for sex drive in both men and women. Some, but not all, researchers believe that testosterone levels decline in men as they age, similar to the way in which estrogen declines in women. The age-related drop in testosterone is called *andropause*. Although controversial, some physicians believe that testosterone-replacement therapy for older men can reverse many of the signs of aging, including loss of muscle and libido.

The quest for a magic potion to increase potency and performance is nothing new. Throughout history, the glands and sexual organs of male animals have been used to create medicines designed to restore potency and increase strength in men. As far back as 3500 years ago, Indian healers recommended using testicular extracts to enhance sexual function in men. Of course, what they didn't know back then was that the testicles contained minute quantities of testosterone. Little research was done on hormones until a now-famous groundbreaking experiment in 1889, performed by Charles Edward Brown Sequard, who injected himself with a blend of extracts from guinea pig and dog testes. Although he reported that the results were nothing short of miraculous, increasing his sex drive and energy, his discovery was considered pure hokum. It wasn't until the 1920s that researchers were able to prove the existence of testosterone, and treating male problems with glandular extracts became quite a fad. Although serious researchers suspected that real testosterone would be an excellent treatment for loss of sex drive and diminished muscle tone that often affected older men, the problem was that there was too little testosterone residue in animal testes to be effective, and therefore, it was essential to develop a way to synthesize the hormone. In 1935, German researchers won the Nobel Prize for creating a synthetic testosterone. In 1945, testosterone captured the imagination of the public with the publication of *The Male Hormone*, by Paul de Kruif, a journalist who was taking testosterone himself, and raved about its positive effects.

Since the discovery of testosterone, there has been a great deal of speculation as to what testosterone actually does and, only recently, have there been any solid, clinical studies. In one 1996 study published in the *New England Journal of Medicine*, researchers reported that testosterone can enhance muscle in men, even if they don't exercise. In the study, which involved male weight lifters, the researchers gave one group of men weekly testosterone injections and another group of men a placebo. Of the men receiving testosterone, one group was put on an exercise program, and one was not. Of the men taking the placebo, one group was put on an exercise program, and one was not. At the end of ten weeks, the testosterone takers had gained more muscle mass than the placebo group, whether they had exercised or not.

Other studies confirm that testosterone has other positive effects on men. It increases energy levels, probably by increasing the level of red blood cells, which provide more oxygen to the body. It also reduces fat, increases lean muscle mass, and improves mood. So, if testosterone is so great, why shouldn't all men take it? Testosterone may cause serious side effects in some men. Although boosting red blood cells gives you energy, excess red blood cells can lead to the formation of blood clots, which can kill you. Testosterone may also lower HDL (good) cholesterol, which can increase the risk of heart disease. And here's a particularly nasty side effect: Testosterone may cause breasts to grow in men, and may stimulate the growth of prostate tumors. There is also a risk that, if you give testosterone to younger men, it will shut down their natural production of testosterone, which will interfere with sexual development and function.

I haven't been able to find any studies that confirm that T-boosters are as effective as testosterone in increasing muscle mass, increasing energy, and enhancing sex drive. Typically, studies of T-boosters have focused on whether the substance actually boosts testosterone at all! These studies are far from conclusive. The main problem is that T-boosters do not uniformly boost testosterone in everyone. In fact, in some cases, they may produce too much estrogen in men, and too much testosterone in women. As discussed in the section on Androstenedione, there have been studies that suggest that T-boosters may offer the disadvantages of testosterone without the advantages. If you use a T-booster, please tell your doctor. You need to be monitored for potential negative side effects.

Possible Benefits

Increase vigor.
Boost libido.
Build muscle.

How to Use It

To get the right dose, work with a knowledgeable physician or natural healer. Remember, any product that is strong enough to significantly boost testosterone needs to be monitored by a doctor.

Cautions

Testosterone is such a hot ticket among body builders, athletes, and both men and women looking for a sexual boost, that many supplements suggest that they boost testosterone when they don't. Overzealous manufacturers have suggested that everything from L-carnitine to yohimbine boosts testosterone. These supplements do other things, but they are *not* T-boosters!

. . . .

TMG

. . . .

 When supplement manufacturers want to breath life into an old product, they'll make a new and exciting claim for it. That's exactly what's happening with TMG, a relatively unknown (and stodgy) supplement that's being spun into a peak performance product. It's being touted as a supplement that can make bigger and stronger muscles. I'm not saying that TMG doesn't work, and, in fact, it may help build muscle, but it does so indirectly. It's also good for your health, especially your heart. (Of course, saying something is heart healthy is not nearly as sexy as promising that it will make you look great!)

So, what is TMG? Also known as *betaine*, TMG is a natural source of methyl groups, molecules consisting of one carbon atom and three hydrogen atoms. TMG is a key player in a process called *methylation*, which is as essential for life as breathing. Methylation is an on-off switch that triggers hundreds of bodily processes. For example, the methylation of protein is critical for the growth and repair for all cells of the body, including muscle cells. The methylation of DNA is also important for cell growth and repair.

Methyl groups are also essential because they help maintain normal levels of *homocysteine*, an amino acid in the body that, at higher than normal levels, has been linked to heart disease, certain forms of cancer and even Alzheimer's disease. In fact, some physicians feel that elevated homocysteine levels are a better predictor of heart disease than cholesterol levels! Methyl groups convert homocysteine into *methionine*, an amino acid which is essential for protein synthesis, necessary to make muscle. Therefore, it may be a bit of a stretch, but not entirely off base, to say that TMG can help build and preserve muscle.

TMG is found in many foods, including broccoli, spinach, and beets.

Possible Benefits

Essential for repair and growth of all cells.

May increase available protein for muscle growth.

How to Use It

The usual dose is 500–1000 mg. daily. I recommend that you take this with 400 mcg. folic acid daily.

TRIBULUS

 Why are body builders and athletes turning to an herb long used in India and China? The buzz is that tribulus can build muscle, boost testosterone, and send your libido into overdrive, at least that's what the manufacturers would like us to believe. Since the herb hit the market in the late 1990s, tribulus has become very popular among body builders and athletes. In fact, it's often included in combination formulas with other testosterone boosters, such as andro and DHEA. Does it work? Studies are scarce, and anecdotal reports are mixed. This is not to say that it doesn't work, simply that, as of yet, the jury is out.

A handful of studies conducted in Eastern Europe and Russia show that tribulus raises levels of LH (luteinizing hormone), which should increase testosterone production in men. One study showed that tribulus did raise blood testosterone levels by 30 percent. Whether this makes tribulus a true anabolic supplement is unclear. There are no studies, however, that link tribulus with an increase in strength or muscle mass. Keep in mind that it is not known whether a temporary boost in testosterone actually stimulates muscle growth. The studies that have shown that testosterone can grow muscle involved daily testosterone supplements given at fairly high doses, over a several-week period. Many experts doubt that an herb would be strong enough to do this without causing the same negative side effects of real testosterone, which include enlargement of the prostate, the growth of breasts in men, and a higher risk for blood clots.

One study conducted in India found that tribulus helped enhance energy and improve mood in men and women suffering from fatigue and mild depression.

Tribulus has long been used as an aphrodisiac and a treatment for infertility. The herb contains steroidallike compounds, such as saponins, which could increase libido.

Guys with prostate problems should steer clear of tribulus or any other substance that boosts testosterone.

Possible Benefits

Boosts energy.
Stimulates libido.

How to Use It

Take two 125 mg. tablets daily.

TYROSINE

facts Feel tired and stressed? Here's a supplement that may help you perform your best in the gym and at the office. *Tyrosine* is a so-called *nonessential amino acid* (meaning that it is produced by the body and need not be obtained through food). It's made from another amino acid, phenylalanine. Trust me, there's nothing nonessential about tyrosine—there are times in your life when you need more tyrosine than your body can make on its own. Tyrosine is key to the production of several *neurotransmitters*, chemical messengers in the brain that help nerves communicate with each other. Neurotransmitters help control mood, concentration, memory, and learning.

Physical and emotional stress can alter the production of neurotransmitters, resulting in physical and mental fatigue. Numerous studies—including some conducted by the U.S. military—have shown that tyrosine supplements taken during times of stress can increase energy levels and relieve the symptoms of mental exhaustion. In particular, studies have demonstrated that tyrosine helps people maintain their mental focus during times of extreme environmental stress, like high altitudes or extremely cold climates. It has also been used to treat chronic fatigue syndrome and depression.

Any supplement that fights both mental and physical fatigue is useful for athletes, particularly those in the midst of a difficult training period. Tyrosine isn't going to pump you up, or make you stronger, but it could give you the stamina to work out longer.

Tyrosine should not be used every day, but only when needed. It raises the levels of the neurotransmitter norepinephrine, which is depleted during times of stress. In excess, norepinephrine can raise blood pressure.

Possible Benefits

Enhances mental function.
Fights fatigue.
Boosts mood.

How to Use It

Take 500 mg. twice daily, or up to an hour before working out. Do not take tyrosine late in the day—it could keep you up at night.

Cautions

Avoid this supplement if you have kidney problems.

VANADIUM

As every body builder knows, insulin shuttles glucose into cells and turns on protein synthesis. This is very important—protein is what builds muscle! *Vanadium* (also called *vanadyl*) is a trace mineral found in food and in our bodies that supposedly mimics the action of insulin. It is a common ingredient in many muscle-building formulas. Although I wasn't able to find any studies verifying that vanadium is a *bona fide* muscle builder, users swear that it helps make them feel really pumped and also speeds recovery. Alas, there is no scientific confirmation!

I have talked with alternative physicians who worry that vanadium (it is most often used in the form of vanadyl sulfate) can cause a rapid decline in blood sugar in some people. So they recommend that it be used with caution and, preferably, under a doctor's supervision. There are no studies to assess its long-term safety. One recent study reported that vanadyl sulfate was useful for people with noninsulin-dependent diabetes mellitis, also known as adult-onset diabetes. One of the reasons people get fat and flabby as they age is that they become insulin resistant—they make plenty of insulin, but their cells no longer respond to it. Insulin resistance is often a result of poor diet and obesity, and can lead to adult-onset diabetes. Insulin resistance is easy to prevent: Exercise, a low-carb diet (only good carbs, minus the refined carbs) and high-quality protein can keep this problem at bay.

Vanadium is found in many foods, including seafood, mushrooms, and soy. You probably get about 15–50 mcg vanadium in your food every day—that's not very much. Vanadium supplements are sold in hefty doses, from 15 mg to 45 mg. If you're using vanadyl sulfate to feed your muscles, be sure to keep within my recommended dose. I think a little goes a long way.

Possible Benefits

May keep glucose under control.
Makes bigger muscles.

How to Use It

Take 15 mg. after working out.

VELVET DEER ANTLER

 This hot, new peak performance supplement is two thousand years old! A scroll uncovered from an ancient tomb in the Hunam province of China lists twenty-two different medical conditions that can be treated with velvet deer antler. Today, this popular Asian remedy is being touted as a muscle builder, sexual revitalizer, and energy booster, as well as an overall rejuvenator. Deer and elk shed their antlers each year and grow new antlers—it is the discarded antlers that are used to make velvet deer antler products. (In other words, no deer or other animals should be harmed in the making of this product!) *Velvet* refers to the soft outside covering on the antler, similar to skin. Once the antler is fully grown, the covering is scrapped off by the animal to sharpen his antlers. The discarded antler reputedly contains special medicinal properties, and is used in Asia to treat a wide variety of ailments.

Russian athletes have reportedly used velvet deer antler to improve performance, strength, and muscle growth. Russian scientists have also reported that athletes who use velvet deer antler recover from their workouts faster. Velvet deer antler may give you more than brawn. At least one study showed that men who took velvet deer antler performed better on mathematical problems than those who did not. It sounds like a lot of hype, but test-tube studies have confirmed that extracts of velvet deer antler contain IGF-1, a hormonal precursor to growth hormone, essential for the growth and maintenance of muscle. Another New Zealand study suggests the velvet deer antler may boost testosterone levels, which will also enhance muscle growth. However, as far as I could find, there is no definitive double-blind, clinical study (the gold standard in the West) linking this supplement to bigger muscles. There is plenty of anecdotal evidence, however, from happy users contending that they get better results from their workout if they take velvet deer antler.

Velvet deer antler is rich in amino acids, collagen, and contains anti-inflammatory substances. In fact, it is a good source of chondroitin sulfate, the arthritis treatment. It's possible that velvet deer antler could help heal and possibly even prevent joint injuries due to overuse or inflammation.

If, as some studies suggest, velvet deer antler increases testosterone levels, it could explain its reputation as a sexual enhancer. (Testosterone regulates sex drive in both men and women.) According to Ron Teeguarden, a leading U.S. authority on Eastern medicine, in Asia it is believed that the bigger the size of the antlers, the more powerful their ability to restore sexual potency. In China, velvet deer antler is considered to be as good a tonic as ginseng. Although velvet deer antler is being promoted as a man's supplement in the West, in Chinese medicine it's been used to treat female menstrual problems and, in general, to promote health and vitality for both sexes.

Velvet deer antler is nontoxic, even at high doses, but Asian physicians do not prescribe it to people with circulatory problems or angina (chest pain.) Although velvet deer antler is used in Asia to treat some forms of heart disease, if you have a heart condition, do not use this supplement unless it is under the supervision of a physician.

Possible Benefits

Energy booster.
Builds muscle.
Relieves inflammation, may be effective against arthritis.
Aphrodisiac and sexual tonic.

How to Use It

Take one 70 mg. capsule daily.

VINPOCETINE

facts
It's being promoted as Viagra for the brain. The newest smart drug to go public is this extract from the periwinkle plant, the same plant that gave us *vincamine*, a potent chemotherapy drug. Vinpocetine is chemically related to caffeine and nicotine, two well-known brain stimulants. However, unlike its better-known relatives, vinpocetine is not addictive. Although it is being mar-

keted as a memory booster for everyone, vincopetine has primarily been used in Europe to treat dementia caused by insufficient blood flow to the brain. It's produced good results in poststroke patients, helping to restore cognitive function. Studies that measure blood flow to the brain have documented that vinpocetine improves cerebral circulation, which means the brain has more nutrients and oxygen. There have been very few studies of vinpocetine, however, on healthy people. One double-blind, crossover study of twelve healthy women (twenty-five to forty years old) compared vinpocetine (at 10 mg., 20 mg., or 40 mg.) to a placebo. On the third day of taking vinpocetine or the placebo, the women were given standard psychological tests to determine cognitive function. After the women took vinpocetine, they showed a dramatic improvement in short-term memory, as opposed to when they took the placebo. There has not been a large, clinical trial of vinpocetine on healthy people to assess its effectiveness. Since vinpocetine has been used for more than twenty years in Europe without problems, it does appear to be safe.

Vinpocetine improves the transport of glucose across the blood–brain barrier, which means that the brain cells have more raw material to make energy. Recent studies reveal that vinpocetine is also an anti-inflammatory. There's a growing body of science that suggests that inflammation in the brain may be a key factor in Alzheimer's disease and normal brain aging. Some researchers believe that the key to preventing the age related loss in brain function may be by controlling inflammation.

A side benefit of vinpocetine—it has been used successfully to treat *tinnitis*, or chronic ringing in the ears, possibly due to poor circulation.

Possible Benefits

Enhances short-term memory.

How to Use It

Although the dose recommended by some manufacturers is as little as 10mg., higher doses, up to 40 mg. daily, may be required.

VITAMIN B-1

 You can't function at your peak if you don't get enough of this B vitamin! Although *beri beri*, a disease caused by a severe B-1 deficiency, is rare in the West, I believe that many people have subclinical B-1 deficiency, robbing them of energy and reducing their mental function. In other words, although it's not making them sick, it is keeping them from performing optimally. In a recent study performed at the University of Wales, 120 healthy women college students were either given 50 mg. B-1 or a placebo. All but one had what would be considered normal levels of B-1 at the beginning of the study. Two months after beginning the vitamin therapy, the women who took B-1 had higher scores on psychological tests checking their reaction time, were in better moods, and more clear-headed than the placebo takers.

Why does B-1 (also called *thiamine*) affect brain function? Vitamin B-1 is essential to process food into energy or ATP, the fuel that runs the body. Your nervous system requires B-1 to work well, too. Alcohol saps the body of B vitamins in general, and B-1 in particular. So does a high-sugar, high-carbohydrate diet. Good food sources of thiamine include rice bran, soybeans, and wheat germ. Because so many of us eat poorly and on the run, I recommend taking a B-complex supplement daily.

Possible Benefits

More energy.
Better mental focus.

How to Use It

Take a multivitamin supplement with B-complex vitamins, including 25–50 mg. B-1.

VITAMIN C

 Since my late friend and dear colleague Linus Pauling first introduced the world to the powers of vitamin C, it's been touted as the cure for the common cold. Recent studies suggest that vitamin C may actually be the cure for *cortisol overload*, that is, for those times when you're pumping too much of the stress hormone that throws you into a catabolic state.

Numerous studies have documented that, although vitamin C can't prevent a cold, it can speed up recovery from a cold. There's a huge concentration of vitamin C in immune cells, which suggests that it plays a role in immunity. In fact, marathon runners who take vitamin C have a lower incidence of respiratory infections than runners who do not. Other studies have shown that exposure to high levels of cortisol can dampen immune function. Now, here's the link between cortisol and vitamin C. The adrenal glands in both humans and animals, which produce stress hormones, also contain high amounts of vitamin C, which suggests that vitamin C also plays a role in the production of stress hormones. Could vitamin C's disease-fighting ability stem from its role as regulator of cortisol? In an experiment conducted at the University of Alabama, researchers gave laboratory rats 200 mg. per day of vitamin C (a dose equivalent to several grams a day in humans). The experiment was designed to see first, how vitamin C would affect the production of *corticosterone*, the rodent version of cortisol and second, whether it would reduce the expected drop in immune function experienced by stressed animals. The researchers stressed the animals by immobilizing them for an hour a day over a three-week period. The rats given vitamin C fared a lot better than the untreated rats subjected to the same experiment. Vitamin C rats not only maintained normal levels of stress hormones, but had stronger immune systems. There was another important difference between the two groups of rats—the stressed-out rats that did not get vitamin C lost more weight than the vitamin C treated rats. Although the researchers did not compare lean tissue in the untreated *versus* treated animals, it's likely that the stressed-out rats that did not receive vitamin C were in a catabolic state where they were burning lean muscle mass, not fat. My hunch is that vitamin C protected the treated rats from losing excess amounts of muscle, which is one of the reasons why anyone who engages in vigorous exercise should take a daily vitamin C supplement.

Vitamin C may also help reduce damage to your joints. Vitamin C is essential for the formation of collagen, necessary for the formation of connective tissue, bones, and blood vessels. People with arthritis—or those of you who beat up your joints with weight-bearing activity—should be sure to take vitamin C.

Possible Benefits

Helps control stress hormones.
Boosts immune function.
Protects against cortisol-induced muscle wasting.

How to Use It

Take 500–1000 mg. vitamin C complex up to twice daily, with food.

VITAMIN E

The focus of the *Peak Performance Bible* is not just on supplements that will enhance your performance today; I am equally concerned about your ability to perform well in the years and decades to come. Many of you are training so hard for short-term gain that you are inadvertently setting yourselves up for health problems down the road. I'm not even talking about the later decades of life—I'm talking about problems that will crop up as early as your thirties and forties! There's nothing that ages you faster than injuries that prevent you from getting enough exercise. The good news is there are simple things that you can do right now to help you maintain a strong body later. Taking an adequate amount of vitamin E is one of the easiest things you can do to protect your body.

Here's why you need it. As you know by now, during vigorous exercise, your oxygen intake increases to accommodate the additional workload. This is good, because it enables us to quickly switch into high gear, but bad because you produce more free radicals.

Several studies have documented that both endurance and strength-training athletes have significantly higher levels of free radicals after intense exercise. In one study of male college students, exhaustive exercise resulted in a sharp increase in serum lipid peroxide levels, a marker for free radicals. Elevated levels of key enzymes indicated free-radical muscle damage. The problem is that if your body needs to expend a great deal of protein and energy repairing damaged muscle, it will not be able to build new muscle. Over time, you will *lose* muscle. When the men were given 300 mg. vitamin E daily for four weeks, however, the levels of free radicals dramatically decreased after exhausting exercise, and their enzyme activity was lower. In other words, vitamin E should help retain muscle. Other studies have shown that athletes have significant skeletal muscle damage (as measured by levels of the intramuscular enzyme *creatine kinase*, a marker of cell damage) after a vigorous workout. What does this have to do with vitamin E? In a study of twelve weight-trained men, levels of creatine kinase activity soared after high-intensity resistance exercise, indicating muscle-cell damage. However, when the group took vitamin E supplements for four weeks, their levels of creatine kinase was much lower twenty-four hours after exercise than men taking a placebo!

There's no question that vitamin E can protect your muscles from free-radical damage and, if you work out hard, you should be taking it. Will vitamin E make you a better athlete? Vitamin E does not appear to affect physical performance, with one exception. Studies suggest that vitamin E may help mountain climbers perform better at high altitudes. So, if mountain climbing is your sport, be vigilant about taking your daily dose of vitamin E.

If you engage in activities that beat up your joints (runners and weight lifters, take note), vitamin E may help prevent arthritis by inhibiting the biological pathway that triggers inflammation.

There is a mountain of evidence linking vitamin E supplements to a reduced risk of heart disease. It is especially good at preventing the oxidation of LDL (bad cholesterol), which can damage your arteries and lead to a heart attack.

Possible Benefits

Protects against exercised-induced free radical damage.

Helps you age better.

Prevents heart disease.

Natural anti-inflammatory.

How to Use It

Take one to two 500 IU of the dry, natural D-alpha tocopheryl succinate capsules daily with food.

• •

WATER

• •

facts Water is essential for life. Don't leave home without it! Keep an extra water bottle in your car, your gym bag, and in your desk. When you go out for your morning run, don't forget your water bottle. Dehydration can sneak up on you, especially in warm weather. Water is the most abundant fluid in the human body, accounting for up to two-thirds of total body weight. You can lose water quickly through sweat. If you want to see just how much water you shed when you exercise in hot weather, weight yourself before and after exercise. Four hours of intense exercise in heat and humidity can result in a loss of ten pounds of water weight! Obviously, you need to replenish fluids to prevent severe dehydration and heat stroke.

Drink a glass or two of water before you exercise. Always bring water with you if you are going to be out exercising for more than twenty minutes. Cool water—not ice cold—is best. Ice-cold water may cause cramping. Drink up, even when you're not thirsty. Thirst is not always a good indication of your body's need for water. Know the signs of dehydration. If you are getting enough water, your urine will be a pale yellow. If your urine turns a dark color, it's a sign of dehydration.

Nutrients and hormones circulate throughout the body *via* water. Water cushions and lubricates joints and prevents friction between bones and ligaments. It is critical for every single bodily function, so don't allow yourself to run dry!

I don't drink tap water. I recommend installing a home-filtering system or drinking bottled water from reputable manufacturers. Try to use water that has undergone reverse osmosis, distillation, or a combination of osmosis and deionization. If you have a home-filtering system, remember it must be maintained periodically.

Remember, caffeinated or alcoholic beverages do not count as water—they are natural diuretics that can promote water loss. Fruit juice and sports drinks are fine but, if you're watching your weight, they can add extra calories. Of course, if you're an endurance athlete, you can use those extra calories.

One caveat—don't gulp down too much water too quickly. It could make you sick to your stomach.

Possible Benefits

You can't live without it!

How to Use It

Drink six to eight glasses of water daily—even more if you are exercising outdoors. An easy way to tell how much water you need per day is to divide your weight by two—that is approximately how many ounces you should be drinking. For example, a 160-pound man who is very physically active should drink eighty ounces (10 glasses) water. Drink a cup of water for every cup of coffee you drink. This will replace the water loss.

WHEY PROTEIN POWDERS

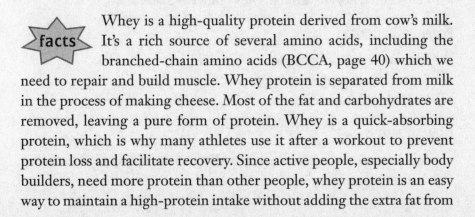

Whey is a high-quality protein derived from cow's milk. It's a rich source of several amino acids, including the branched-chain amino acids (BCCA, page 40) which we need to repair and build muscle. Whey protein is separated from milk in the process of making cheese. Most of the fat and carbohydrates are removed, leaving a pure form of protein. Whey is a quick-absorbing protein, which is why many athletes use it after a workout to prevent protein loss and facilitate recovery. Since active people, especially body builders, need more protein than other people, whey protein is an easy way to maintain a high-protein intake without adding the extra fat from food sources. Whey protein isolate, the most expensive form of whey, contains a higher percentage of protein than whey protein concentrate. Some body builders and professional athletes swear by the isolate, but others say the less pricier concentrate works fine. As far as I'm concerned, both are high-quality proteins. If you feel that you need every conceivable advantage to achieve your goals, and you can afford it, by all means use the isolate! Otherwise, the concentrate is fine.

The benefits of whey protein extend far beyond bigger muscles. Studies show that whey protein can raise blood levels of *glutathione*, a critical antioxidant depleted during strenuous exercise. This is important because glutathione is essential for a healthy immune system. Whey also contains several immunoglobulins and other milk proteins that boost immune function. In fact, whey protein is effective against both salmonella and streptococcus pneumonia infections.

Some manufacturers offer a hydrolyzed or predigested form of whey that may be broken down more rapidly in the gut. It probably is absorbed more rapidly and, once again, if you're looking for every competitive edge, and are willing to pay the price, go ahead and buy the highest-quality protein around.

By the way, I'm not suggesting that whey protein is essential to athletic success. Long before protein powders were available, lots of people achieved amazing results just on food and training alone. I view whey protein as a convenience food for athletes who are necessarily careful about getting enough protein in their diet, and are perfectly happy to down a protein shake or two as insurance against protein loss.

Remember the sonnet, Little Miss Muffet sat on her tuffet eating her curds and whey? Nothing is new under the sun.

Possible Benefits

May stem the loss of protein after workout.
Speeds recovery from exercise.
Helps build muscle.

How to Use It

Mix one to two tablespoons (15–25 grams) whey protein powder daily in liquid.

WHITE WILLOW

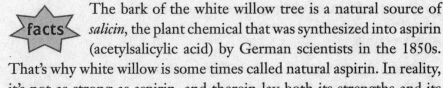

The bark of the white willow tree is a natural source of *salicin*, the plant chemical that was synthesized into aspirin (acetylsalicylic acid) by German scientists in the 1850s. That's why white willow is some times called natural aspirin. In reality, it's not as strong as aspirin, and therein lay both its strengths and its weaknesses.

For centuries, white-willow bark has been used to treat fevers, inflammation, and muscle aches and pains. Today, white willow is being promoted as a thermogenic agent and is often stacked with ephedra and caffeine, or a caffeine source, such as guarana or kola. In this regard, it's riding on the coattails of aspirin. Studies have documented that aspirin can enhance the fat-burning effect of ephedra and caffeine, although some researchers dispute whether the effect of the stack is all that it's cracked up to be. Since white willow is so close in chemical structure to aspirin, some manufacturers claim that it can be used instead of aspirin, in combination with ephedra and caffeine. Unfortunately, there are no studies to verify this claim.

White willow is also used as a treatment for arthritis, although I think there are more effective treatments available, such as MSM and glucosamine/chondroitin.

Some herbalists claim that white willow is as effective as aspirin but without negative side effects like stomach upset, ulcers, or stomach bleeding. I'm not entirely convinced. If taken at high enough doses, white willow could at least theoretically cause the same gastrointestinal problems as aspirin in highly sensitive people. However, unlike aspirin, white willow contains tannins and flavonoids which could be soothing to the stomach. However, I still think it's wise for people with ulcers or an irritable digestion to steer clear of both aspirin and white willow. If you don't have such problems, I believe white willow is a safer choice. In addition, keep in mind that traditional healers prescribed white willow to be used occasionally, not every day. Therefore, I think it is unwise to take this herb as you would a vitamin pill.

Possible Benefits

May enhance fat-burning effects of ephedra and caffeine.
Reduces fever, good for aches and pains of colds.

How to Use It

Take 60–120 mg. of a standardized salicin extract for symptoms.
Thermogenic daily formulas typically contain around 75 mg. of
white willow.

Caution

Because white willow is so similar to aspirin, some herbalists feel it
should not be given to children with fevers. Aspirin can cause Reyes
Syndrome in children with flu or other viruses.

YOHIMBE

 When I first wrote about yohimbe in *Earl Mindell's Supplement Bible*, I said that it was so hot that it was practically walking off the shelves at natural food stores. Back then, it was being touted as a sexual tonic that could enhance libido, energy, and sexual performance in men and women. I know of at least one health-food store in Manhattan where the manager had to keep the yohimbe under lock and key to prevent it from falling into the hands of teenage boys. (Lord knows why they need it, anyway!) Today, I want to tell you about a potential, new application for yohimbe that's going to really excite women: Yohimbe may prove to be the magic bullet for cellulite, those annoying and unflattering fat deposits that appear on thighs and buttocks.

Yohimbe is an extract from the African herb *Corynathe yohimbe*. Yohimbe is a natural fat burner and the good news is that it seems to target cellulite. Yohimbe antagonizes the alpha-2 receptors on fat cells. Alpha-2 fat receptors inhibit fat burning; alpha-3 receptors speed up fat burning. Needless to say, there are lots of alpha-2 receptors on a woman's hips, thighs, and buttocks. (Men don't have as much fat in those areas, therefore, they don't have as many fat receptors.) Yohimbe turns off the alpha-2 fat receptors which, in turn, accelerates fat burning. Theoretically, yohimbe should help eliminate cellulite from these targeted areas. At least one leading sports-supplement manufacturer is testing a yohimbe-based product on women to see if it works. We're following this story closely!

Yohimbe is still selling briskly as a sex-enhancing supplement. A stronger version of yohimbe, *yohimbine hydrochloride*, is an FDA-approved drug for erectile dysfunction. Since the arrival of the prescription drug Viagra, yohimbine has been put on the back burner. Smart manufacturers have now begun touting yohimbe as an herbal Viagra, (often in combination formulas also containing arginine). Yohimbe is not for everybody. It should not be used by people with kidney disease, pregnant or nursing women, or anyone with high blood pressure, or anxiety attacks. In fact, at normal doses, although rare, some people can experience dizziness and rapid heart beat, among other problems. So, do be careful. Frankly, if you use yohimbe, I prefer that you work with a medical professional. The buzz is that a safer version of this herb will be available soon.

Recently, yohimbe has also been used to treat depression in people who are nonresponsive to serotonin reuptake inhibitors, such as Prozac.

Possible Benefits

Increases the burning of fat.
Anticellulite.
Enhances sex drive and performance.

How to Use It

Take one to three 500 mg. tablets or capsules daily.

Caution

When taking yohimbe, avoid eating foods with high amounts of tyrosine, including cheese, red wine, and liver. It could cause a sudden rise in blood pressure.

ZINC

 During times of intense training, you need more zinc! A recent study of cyclists examined the relationship between overtraining and zinc depletion, and the possible effect of zinc deficiency on health and endurance. In the study, one group of cyclists worked out every day, while another group of cyclists took two to three days a week off from their training regimen. The researchers then measured the amount of zinc lost in the sweat of both groups of cyclists. They found that those who exercised daily lost zinc at a much faster rate than those who didn't push themselves as hard. The loss of zinc has potentially serious consequences. Zinc is a very important mineral for the growth and repair of cells. It is also critical for immune function. It's well known that athletes who are pushing themselves to the limit frequently suffer from respiratory infections, as well as excessive fatigue and decreased stamina. Researchers speculate the loss of zinc could be one factor that is draining these athletes of their strength and leaving them vulnerable to every bug that comes their way.

Recently, zinc has been touted as a sex-enhancing mineral for men and is included in many combination formulas for male sexual performance. There is some truth to this. Zinc is essential for testosterone production, but taking supplemental zinc is not going to send your testosterone levels soaring. It may produce a mild boost, if any. There are also high levels of zinc in the male prostate gland. Moreover, zinc supplementation has been shown to boost sperm count in men with fertility problems. Interestingly, oysters, which have long been touted as a male aphrodisiac, are rich in zinc!

The older you are, the more zinc you need. Marginal zinc deficiency is widespread among people over fifty. Zinc is especially important to maintain a strong immune system but, if you exercise on a regular basis, be vigilant about getting enough zinc. Good food sources of zinc include pumpkin seeds, brewer's yeast, wheat germ, pork, and beans.

Possible Benefits

Can assist recovery from workout.

Important to prevent exercise-induced decline in immunity.

May enhance fertility in men.

How to Use It

Take 15–60 mg. zinc daily.

. . . .

ZMA

. . . .

facts   Zinc magnesium aspartate (ZMA) is being marketed as a new and improved form of zinc that can safely boost testosterone levels without the side effects associated with anabolic steroids, the andros or DHEA. Does it work? In one study performed at Western Washington University, in Bellingham, it lived up to its reputation. In this study, a group of college football players took either ZMA or a placebo for eight weeks. The group that took ZMA showed a significant boost in free testosterone levels versus the placebo users, as well as an increase in muscle strength. It would be nice to see more studies duplicating these good results.

Among the general population, few people get the full RDA for either zinc or magnesium everyday. Due to the greater demands placed on their bodies, athletes may even have deficits in these essential minerals. In addition, even minor deficiencies in these minerals may hamper testosterone production and compromise immune function.

ZMA isn't going to turn you into a superman, but it contains minerals that are basically safe and good for you, as long as you don't exceed the recommended dose. It's a lot safer than messing around with hormones! It's especially good for teen athletes who eat poorly and are more likely to suffer nutritional deficiencies.

Zinc is also an immune booster that is essential for the production of disease fighting T-cells. ZMA may help keep you healthier.

Possible Benefits

May increase testosterone levels.
May enhance muscle strength.
Immune booster.

How to Use It

The recommended dose varies among manufacturers. The typical daily dose ranges from 45–90 mg. zinc and 1000–1200 mg. magnesium.

Caution

Too much magnesium can give you diarrhea and an upset stomach, especially if you're prone to such problems. If you have an irritable stomach, proceed with caution. Start with a low dose, then work your way up. If it causes stomach upset, don't use it!

3

PEAK PERFORMANCE NUTRITION

When it comes to performing at your peak, the right diet can make the difference between staying on top of your game, and failing to achieve your goals. There is no pill or potion—legal or otherwise—that can compensate for poor nutrition or a sedentary lifestyle. Eating wisely will help create sleek muscles and a well-toned body, as well as providing the strength and stamina you need to make it through the long haul. The supplements that I recommend in this book can help enhance your performance, but they can't do the job alone.

It sounds so simple—eat well and you'll look terrific, feel great, and perform at your peak. The problem is, when it comes to food, there is a lot of confusion and misinformation. Despite the fact that dieting has become a national pasttime, Americans are fatter than ever. Obesity is a major health crisis for both adults and children. Eating disorders among both women and men have become a national epidemic. In fact, in the name of fitness, many of you are harming yourselves by adhering to fad diets that rob your body of vital nutrients and leave you vulnerable to disease in your later decades. The consumption of junk food is soaring. According to the National Cancer Institute, one-third to one-half of all cancers may be due to poor diet. Shockingly, only 25 percent of Americans are eating what they should to prevent cancer! Heart disease, which is the number one killer of both men and women, is also linked to poor diet, as are diabetes and osteoporosis. As I like to remind people, the body you have today is going to have to sustain you throughout the rest of your life. You have a choice. You can maintain it well, or you can run it into the ground.

In this chapter, I will provide the basic information you need to eat to win while, at the same time, maintaining a strong, healthy body today, tomorrow, and in the years to come. I know that many of you are at different levels of fitness. Some of you may be trying to shed a few pounds; others may be in great shape and trying to stay that way. The truth is, the rules of good nutrition are the same no matter who you are. Granted, if you work out vigorously every day, you will need more food than someone who is sedentary. Someone who is preparing for a marathon may eat differently before an event than a weight lifter. However, there are basic truths about nutrition that apply to everyone. Once you arm yourself with the right information, you will be in a better position to make the right food choices for you.

Think Macro

Macronutrients are nutrients that provide us with energy—protein, carbohydrate, and fat. Macronutrients are ingested in much larger quantities than *micronutrients*—vitamins, minerals, and other chemicals from food that we need to maintain heath. Without micronutrients, we could not digest macronutrients.

In recent years, there has been a great deal of controversy over which macronutrient is most important. So-called experts have told us to cut back on protein and fat and load up on carbs; others have preached the virtues of all protein and no carbs; still others have told us to eat more fat. It's all so confusing! The fact is, all of the macronutrients are important; they each perform different jobs in the body.

All About Protein

Protein is essential for the normal growth and maintenance of body tissues. Every system of the body, from the heart to the endocrine system (which makes hormones), depends on adequate amounts of protein. You also need protein to build muscle!

In your body, protein is broken down into amino aids, which combine in various ways to form the cells and tissues of the body. There are twenty-two different amino acids. The essential amino acids cannot be made by the body and must be obtained through food. They include isoleucine, leucine, lysine, methionine, phenylalanine, threonine, tryptophan, and valine. Six of the amino acids are *nonessential*, which means they are made by the body and need not be obtained through food. These include alanine, asparagine, aspartic acid, glutamic acid, glycine and serine. (Even though alanine is considered nonessential, some athletes may need more of it than their bodies can make. See page 22.) Seven of the amino acids are called *conditionally* essential, which means that they may be essential under certain circumstances. (For example, histadine is not essential for adults, but is considered essential for infants and small children.)

Milk, eggs, dairy, fish, poultry and other animal products contain all eight essential fatty acids. With the exception of protein found in soy foods and a handful of grains (quinoa, spelt, and triticale) plant foods do not contain all the essential amino acids. If you are a vegetarian who eats dairy and eggs, it is easier to get all the amino acids you need than if you only eat foods derived from plants.

Vegetarians should eat complementary proteins—foods that, if consumed together, contain all eight essential amino acids. For example, the amino acids found in grains are different from those found in legumes, but if you eat grains and legumes together (like a dish of rice and beans) you have a complete protein. Vegetarians can be very healthy, but it does take some thought. Many teenagers are attracted to vegetarianism and, since they're bodies are still growing, it is imperative that they know the right way to eat. If you don't get enough body-building amino acids, you cannot perform at your best.

Your daily protein requirement will vary according to activity level. The RDI (Recommended Daily Intake) for protein is .8 grams of protein per kilogram of body weight, or .36 grams per pound. By those figures, a 150-pound man would need about 54 grams of protein daily. However, endurance and strength athletes may require significantly more (1–1.6 grams per pound of body weight) or 25 to 30 percent of total daily calories. Ironically, most sedentary Americans consume way too much protein for their activity level, while many athletes consume too little. Remember, if you eat a lot of protein and don't work it off, it will be converted into fat. If you work out hard, however, it may help build muscle. Some studies suggest that ingesting high amounts of protein if you do serious resistance training can increase muscle size and strength.

What about very high-protein diets (for example, Atkins and Protein Power) whereby you eat massive amounts of protein along with some vegetables, and virtually no grains and very little fruit? It's true that people who can stick to such a strict diet lose weight, often rapidly. However, much of that is water weight. Carbohydrates hold onto to water (which is why people rehydrate with carbohydrate-rich sports drinks after working out). As soon as you begin eating carbs again, you will put back the weight. Therein lies the problem. Very few people can stay on a high-protein, very-low-carb diet for any length of time. It's really boring! Excess protein can be harmful for people with kidney problems. So . . . I don't think highly restrictive diets are the best way to achieve permanent weight loss. I also believe that by eliminating entire categories of food, you are denying yourself important disease-fighting nutrients that I'll talk about later.

The Best Sources of Protein

Protein comes in many different packages—some better for you than others. The rule of thumb is that all animal protein has about 7 grams of protein per ounce. That means ounce for ounce, fish, turkey, red meat, and eggs contain the same amount of protein. Three ounces of animal protein is equal in size to a standard deck of cards. So why does three ounces of steak make you feel fuller than three ounces of fish? In most cases, red meat contains more fat than most types of fish, and fat helps you feel more full. Although some forms of fat are better than others, too much fat can increase your risk of heart disease and cancer—not to mention the fact that fat is very fattening (9 calories per gram of fat *versus* 4 calories per gram of protein). When you select your protein source, consider its fat content. (For more information on how to tell good fats from bad fats, see page 181.)

Generally, leaner forms of protein are preferable to high-fat varieties, and that goes for everybody, including those of you who need to take off weight, as well as those of you who are at your ideal weight, but want to put on more muscle. The guys and gals at the gym with super-cut bodies are not gorging on high-fat cheeseburgers or fried chicken! They're eating chicken breast or turkey (I bet without the skin), leaner cuts of beef (like flank steak or London broil), soybean veggie burgers, hard-boiled eggs, and grilled fish (like salmon or tuna) over greens. Those who don't like to cook or who eat on the run are grabbing high-quality protein shakes, not junk food. And they're washing their meals down with filtered water, not soda.

Proteins to Avoid

Although many of the popular high-protein diets do not distinguish between the various forms of protein, I feel very strongly that there are protein foods that should be avoided. In particular, I urge you to pass on processed meats (hot dogs, salami, bologna, sausage, and bacon). These meats are not only laden with bad fat, but contain nitrites, chemicals that are converted into carcinogenic substances in the gut. People who consume high amounts of these foods may be increasing their risk of stomach cancer. Bacon and sausage lovers, don't despair. Canadian bacon contains less fat than regular bacon, although it can still contain nitrites. If you look hard enough, you may be able to find a nitrite-free Canadian bacon at a natural food supermarket or gourmet butcher. Alternative sausage (made from chicken, mushroom, soy) that is preservative-free can be found at many enlightened supermarkets and natural food stores. Many brands are delicious, and can be seasoned with pine nuts, sun-dried tomatoes and other really tasty stuff. (In other words, you don't have to feel sorry for yourself—feel sorry for the other guy eating nitrites who may get cancer in twenty years!)

Whenever possible, I recommend that you use hormone-free,

antibiotic-free poultry and meat. You want your body to expend its energy on getting stronger, not on fighting the effects of unnecessary toxins. You can find these products easily at a well-stocked supermarket or natural food store. When it comes to fish, pollution is also an issue. Obviously, don't eat fish if you know that it's been caught in polluted waters. Farm-raised fish is good because it is pollutant free.

The Carbohydrate Controversy

Carbohydrate is a general term for a wide range of foods with seemingly little in common, ranging from soda to whole grains to chips to fresh fruits to candy bars to vegetables. Carbohydrates include sugars and starches that, during digestion, are broken down in the body into *glucose*, a simple sugar used to make energy. Carbohydrate that is not immediately used by the body is stored as glycogen in muscles and the liver. If the glycogen is not used up, it's converted into fat.

Carbohydrates are the body's main source of energy. If you work out hard, you need to have enough stored glycogen on hand to fuel your workout. If you don't have enough glycogen, you will tire easily and be unable to perform well. That's why endurance athletes load up on carbohydrates (so-called carbo loading) days before a major event—they know that if they run out of glycogen, they will run out of steam. Exercising for two hours straight or running twenty miles will deplete your glycogen stores. Immediately following a hard training session or a race, savvy athletes know to replenish their glycogen levels by eating a light carbohydrate meal or drinking a carbohydrate-rich beverage.

During times of intense training athletes may require up to 70 percent of their total calories in the form of carbohydrates (roughly 4.5 grams per day of carbohydrate per pound of body weight). If you're not as active, you may need somewhat less, but you still need a fair amount of carbohydrate.

Recently, however, there have been a slew of diets that claim that carbohydrates are fattening and that the answer to permanent weight loss is to eat as few of them as possible. This is only half true. The truth is that some carbohydrates are fattening and, if you're trying to lose weight or maintain your weight, they are definitely off limits. However, there are real differences among the quality of carbohydrates. In other words, there are some carbohydrates that are good for you, and some that are just plain bad. You need to understand the difference and exercise common sense.

Good Carbs, Bad Carbs

There are two different types of carbohydrate—simple and complex. *Simple carbohydrates* are chemically designed to break down very rapidly in the bloodstream, causing a sharp rise in sugar. Simple carbohydrates generally include sugar-laden foods, such as refined, processed grain products; soda; candy; highly sweetened cereals; undiluted juices; and cookies. The problem with these foods is that they get burned up too fast which, before too long, can leave you hungry for more. Sugar triggers a rise in the hormone insulin, which is not necessarily bad—insulin promotes the production and storage of glucose and fat, and increases protein production. When you eat a lot of simple carbohydrates, however, you get frequent insulin spikes, leading to equally rapid drops in insulin. This is what makes you feel tired, hungry, and cranky. If you eat even more simple carbohydrates (like a candy bar and a can of sweetened ice tea), you'll begin to see that those excess carbohydrate calories will be stored as fat. There is also the potential for long-term damage. Some scientists believe that a high-sugar diet can lead to a condition known as *insulin resistance* which, in turn, can lead to Type II diabetes. In Type II diabetes, you make plenty of insulin, but your cells don't respond to it. This can lead to obesity, muscle wasting, and heart disease.

Soda is a particularly bad culprit—you can guzzle gallons of the stuff and not even realize that you are loading up on bad carbohydrates and sugar. The consumption of soda has skyrocketed in the United States—the average person drinks fifty-five gallons of carbonated soft drinks a year (that's more than milk, fruit juice, and bottled water combined!)

Complex carbohydrates, which are broken down more slowly in the blood stream, are a better food choice. They include whole grains, legumes (beans), and most fruits and vegetables. Complex carbohydrates contain fiber, which slows the breakdown of carbohydrates in the blood. Fiber is very important for health. It helps to maintain bowel regularity, can lower high cholesterol, and appears to protect against insulin resistance. Fiber is rich in the mineral *magnesium*, which protects against diabetes and heart disease, and *phytic acid*, which may protect against cancer and help regulate blood sugar. Fiber also makes you feel full, so you're not apt to eat as much. Some high-protein–low-carbohydrate diets are so deficient in fiber that people are advised to use laxatives. To me, this is ridiculous. It's a sign that you're not eating the way nature intended you to eat. Throw out those laxatives and start eating some real fiber!

Not all complex carbohydrates get my seal of approval. Another factor to consider is the *glycemic index* (GI), which rates foods according to how they affect blood sugar levels. The GI was developed by David Jenkin, Ph.D., for diabetics who need to avoid sugar surges. Recently, some physicians have begun recommending it to their patients as a means of preventing diabetes, and as a possible weight-loss tool. In fact, some studies have linked a steady diet of high GI meals with obesity.

Many complex carbohydrates score well on the GI. The best performers are most green vegetables, lentils and other legumes, rice and pasta (cooked *al dente*), oranges, sweet potatoes, and pumpernickel bread. In fact, with few exceptions, starchy foods (breads and cereals) cause a greater increase in blood sugar than do fresh vegetables. To be on the safe side, I recommend that you limit your intake of starchy foods to no more than two to three servings daily. (One serving equals one slice of bread, or half cup cereal, pasta, or rice.) Cherries and berries, which score well for fruit, are also terrific sources of other good vitamins and nutrients that can keep you healthy. White bread and white rice don't score well, but I don't think they have much food value anyway. Brown rice is far better in terms of its GI rating and nutrient content. Steel-cut oatmeal is a better choice than instant oatmeal, which makes sense; it's less processed. Bananas, beets, carrots, corn, and white potatoes should be eaten in limited quantities, because they raise blood-sugar levels so dramatically. There are some oddities on the GI—potato chips actually score better than whole-wheat bread, which contains fiber, B vitamins, and other important nutrients. There is no way I would advise anyone to eat potato chips over whole wheat bread! What the GI doesn't take into account is that potato chips contain fats called *transfatty acids*, which are bad for your heart. So, as with anything else, the GI is a useful guide, but should not be followed slavishly.

As good as complex carbohydrates may be, you should not eat them without some protein. Protein and fat helps stabilize blood-sugar levels and will prevent you from feeling hungry all the time.

Facts About Fat

For most people, about 15 to 20 percent of daily calories should be in the form of fat. I know that some diets suggest that 30 percent of daily calories should come from fat, but considering the fact that fat is so calorie dense, I don't think that's a good idea.

Not that very low-fat diets work, either! Diets that restrict you to 10 percent fat are difficult to follow, and tend to be tasteless. You do need some fat to survive. Fat is essential for hormone production, and to maintain cell membranes, the outer covering of every cell. The gray matter of your brain is very high in fat. Extremely low-fat diets often result in fatigue, dry skin and hair, brittle nails, constant hunger, and even depression. Ironically, very low-fat diets make you lose muscle and gain weight! The trick is to choose the right fats.

There are three types of fat: saturated fat, monounsaturated fat, and polyunsaturated fat:

Saturated fat is found primarily in animal sources (meat, eggs, dairy). It has been linked to an increased risk of heart disease because it can raise blood cholesterol levels.

Monounsaturated fat is abundant in common cooking oils (like olive oil and canola oil). This fat contains antioxidants and is believed to protect against heart disease.

Polyunsaturated fat is found in vegetable oils (safflower, corn, and sunflower) and margarine. They can be good . . . or they can be bad.

Here's where it gets a bit confusing. On the surface, polyunsaturated fats seem to be healthy. However, when polyunsaturated fats are hardened, in a process called *hydrogenation*, this creates transfatty acids, which can raise blood cholesterol levels and may increase the risk of breast cancer. Some, but not all brands of margarine contain transfatty acids. If you use margarine, buy only transfatty-acid-free margarine. (Personally, I prefer a little olive oil or a small amount of butter.) The problem is that transfatty acids are hidden throughout the food supply, and are especially abundant in processed foods. Unfortunately, food manufacturers don't have to tell consumers the amount of transfatty acids in processed foods. The FDA is now considering changing the labeling requirements to include transfatty acids. I don't need to read a label—if a food is processed or fried, it probably contains transfatty acids.

Most people get plenty of bad fat, but not enough good fat. In particular, our diets are lacking a type of polyunsaturated fat called *omega-3 fatty* acids. Omega-3s are found in fatty fish (salmon, tuna, mackerel, sardines), eggs from specially fed chickens, and some grains and seeds. Our hunter-gatherer ancestors ate a diet that was much richer in omega-3 fatty acids than we do, and some scientists believe that many of our modern diseases, from cancer to heart disease to depression, are, in part a result of an omega-3 fatty acid deficiency.

Omega-3 fatty acids contain alpha linolenic acid, which is metabolized in the body into EPA (eicosapentaoic acid) and DHA (docosahexaenoic acid). DHA, in particular, is believed to be especially important for the maintenance of the brain. In fact, a diet low in DHA has been linked to an increased risk of depression. You need to eat two to three servings of fatty fish weekly to maintain the right levels of DHA. For those of you don't eat fish, flaxseed is also an excellent source of omega-3 fatty acids. Ground flaxseed is sold in natural food stores. Sprinkle two tablespoons on cereal, yogurt, fruit, or in a protein shake for an extra omega-3 charge.

The Micronutrients

The current popular diets tend to fixate on the macronutrients. Well-known diet doctors can debate for hours over the correct percentages of protein, fat, and carbohydrates in the body. Sometimes I feel that these so-called experts are missing the forest for the trees! For one thing, these discussions rarely touch upon the quality of food, which I feel is every bit as important as the macronutrient content. If your protein choices are high-fat meats laden with bad chemicals (like luncheon meats) then you are doing yourself even more harm than eating a healthy carbohydrate (like whole grains). Furthermore, few of these diet gurus discuss the importance of micronutrients—vitamins, minerals, and other chemicals found in food. In reality, without micronutrients, the body could not make energy, or perform any of its basic functions, let alone perform at its peak. That's why I feel it is of vital importance for you to understand the importance of incorporating the right amount of micronutrients in your diet.

In order to make sure that you are getting all the necessary vitamins and minerals, I recommend that you take a high-potency multivitamin/mineral supplement daily. Look for one containing a variety of antioxidants (like vitamin C, E, selenium), B-complex, and minerals such as magnesium (500 mg.) and calcium (1000 mg.). (Calcium is particularly important for athletes—it can help prevent muscle cramps!) Teenagers and premenopausal women may need a multivitamin containing iron, particularly if they engage in endurance sports. However, men and postmenopausal women should avoid iron unless it is prescribed by their physicians or natural healer.

Know Your Phytochemicals

In addition to the well-known vitamins and minerals, there is growing evidence that special substances found in plants, called *phytochemicals*, may also help prevent disease and maintain optimal health. Many phytochemicals have strong antioxidant action, which will help you recover faster from your workout, as well as preventing many degenerative diseases. Most of the important phytochemicals are in the pigments of plants. Dark-green vegetables have different phytochemicals than bright orange or yellow fruits and vegetables. Therefore, you need to eat a variety of different colored food to get the full benefits nature has to offer. Here is a list of power foods that are particularly good sources of important phytochemicals.

APPLES. Apples are a great source of fiber, have a good GI score, and contain antioxidant flavonoids. They are light enough to eat before your workout for a quick pick-me-up without weighing you down. Keep one in your gym bag at all times!

ASIAN MUSHROOMS. Asian mushrooms (shiitake, reishi, maitake, and enoki) contain *beta glucans*, special phytochemicals that help keep your immune system strong. Chop a mixture of mushrooms and saute them in a stir fry; throw dried shiitake mushrooms in soup. Look for these special mushrooms at natural food stores and the larger supermarket chains, or order them at Asian restaurants. They're also packed with fiber.

BLUEBERRIES. These berries are a great source of *anthocyanidins*, potent antioxidants that may offer special protection against brain aging. Throw a handful of berries in your protein shake, or sprinkle them in your cereal or over plain yogurt. (Black raspberries, which can be quite pricey, are also a great source of anthocyanidins.)

CHERRIES. A great way to satisfy your sweet tooth without sending your blood sugar into overdrive. Cherries contain *ellagic acid*, a cancer fighter.

GREENS. Dark-green leafy vegetables (watercress, Swiss chard, collard greens, mustard greens, and beet greens) pack a powerful antioxidant punch. In particular, they contain important carotenoids such as lutein and zeaxanthin, which may protect against *macular degeneration*, a leading cause of blindness. If you exercise outdoors a great deal, your eyes are exposed to UV sun rays, which contribute to both cataracts and macular degeneration. Eating a serving of dark greens daily may help to preserve your vision. (Whenever possible, do wear sunglasses!)

ORANGES. A great portable snack! Low on the GI scale, oranges contain a cancer-fighting compound called *limonoid* in the white pulp between sections.

RED GRAPES. Red grapes contain compounds called *polyphenols*, antioxidants that prevent the oxidation of LDL, bad cholesterol. Red grapes are great in salads or eaten alone. (I prefer whole grapes to grape juice because whole grapes contain fiber, juice doesn't.)

SPICES. Spices such as turmeric, ginger, rosemary, and cayenne not only add intense flavor to your food, but are a great source of antioxidants. Also, I think they keep you from overeating. Here's why. I think many people overeat because they're bored with their food. Satisfying your taste buds with a blast of flavor may make you less likely to reach for seconds or thirds.

STRAWBERRIES. These sweet fruits are a great combination of fiber, ellagic acid, and vitamin C. Throw a few in your morning protein shake.

TOMATO. Think *lycopene*, a carotenoid that may protect against both prostate and skin cancer. Also, think great skin—carotenoids appear to help protect the skin from damaging UV rays. (Cooked tomato mixed with olive oil releases lycopene in a form that is absorbable by the body.)

SALAD BAR VEGGIES. Lunch or dinner from a well-stocked salad bar is a terrific and easy way to get your phytochemicals. Pass over the anemic looking iceberg lettuce, and fill your plate with broccoli and cauliflower (they contain cancer-fighting indoles), onion (it contains the antioxidant selenium), yellow and red peppers (great sources of carotenoids), artichoke hearts (lowers cholesterol), tomato (you know why!), and maybe a piece or two of cooked tofu (rich in *isoflavones*, hormonelike chemicals in plants that mimic the action of hormones in the body without the negative side effects). Only patronize salad bars that have fresh food and appear to follow good hygiene. Food that is overhandled or left out too long can become a breeding ground for bacteria.

WALNUTS. Rich in essential fatty acids, walnuts also contain ellagic acid and are a good source of protein. Try sprinkling some over a salad with chunks of cold, chopped chicken breast, sliced apple, and grapes (a modified Waldorf salad). For a quick snack, pack a handful of walnuts in a plastic bag and munch on them when you're hungry. For a healthy lunch on the run, add an apple and wash it down with a cup of soy milk. Remember, walnuts are high in calories, so a little goes a long way.

Tips For a Peak Performance Body

DRINK UP! Drink eight to ten glasses of filtered water daily. Divide your weight by two; this will equal approximately how many ounces of water you need per day. For example, for a 154-pound man, divide 154 by two, which equals 77 ounces, which is about ten (eight-ounce) glasses of water daily. A 125-pound woman would need about sixty-two ounces of water or eight (eight-ounce) glasses daily. If you exercise to the point that you're sweating, add another glass or two to your total!

AVOID HIDDEN CALORIES IN DRINKS. Two glasses of soda (250 calories), one glass of sweetened ice tea (70 calories), two glasses of wine (200 calories). By the end of the day, you could be consuming 500 calories (probably 20 to 25 percent of your ideal caloric intake) in the form of beverages. Which goes back to my first tip—stick to water as much as possible.

READ LABELS CAREFULLY. If one serving of a food product contains more than 20 percent fat and sugar (carbohydrates) or too much sodium (your daily sodium intake should be under 3000 mg.), don't buy it. This should save you about 25 percent on your grocery bill.

COUNT NUTRIENTS, NOT CALORIES. Don't become obsessive about counting calories. I have found that if you concentrate on a nutrient-dense, healthy diet packed with the right foods, you will be more satisfied and will eat less.

BECOME A MINDFUL EATER. Don't eat while watching television, in a moving vehicle, standing up, or at a movie. This is called *unconscious eating*, which causes you to overeat beyond your satiation level. Just watch people eating popcorn at a movie theater! They're shoveling it in without giving it a thought.

DON'T GROCERY SHOP WHEN YOU'RE HUNGRY. If you do, you will buy high-calorie, low-fiber, high-sugar comfort foods that are low in nutrition. Consider your grocery store to be a battle zone. The staples are located in the rear, around the perimeter of the store. The middle aisles and the checkout stand are piled high with impulse items that are high-profit, mostly processed, foods (like sugary cereals and sodas) and junk foods. Have you ever considered that, in the larger supermarkets, they have a small area for health foods? What does that say about the other foods they sell?

RIDE THE WAVE. Remember, hunger comes in waves. Don't go racing out to eat at the first hunger pang. Chances are, it will pass. Wait until you are really hungry to eat.

KNOW WHEN TO STOP. Of equal importance is knowing when to stop. Get in touch with your body. Use this hunger scale: one is famished, five is comfortable, and ten is stuffed. Hold your hand on your stomach and determine where you are on the hunger scale. Stay at five to six if you want to lose weight. Go to seven to ten to gain weight.

SAUCES AND DRESSING ON THE SIDE. You don't have to eat dried-out food, but you shouldn't drown your salad or entrees in high-calorie dressing or sauce. My solution? Ask for your dressing and sauce on the side. Dip each piece of salad or meat in a small amount of dressing or sauce. You'll use about one-tenth the amount, without sacrificing taste.

MAKE FUNCTIONAL EXERCISE A WAY OF LIFE. You don't have to work out at a gym to get exercise. Make a concerted effort to move during the day. Park your car as far away from where you work, live, or shop as possible and walk as much as you can. If you can walk briskly, just two miles per day (about forty city blocks), you can lose about half a pound per week or twenty-six pounds per year.

Peak Performance Nutrition Tips
For Your Kids

The statistics tell the story—American kids are getting fatter and fatter. Thirteen percent of all American kids are seriously overweight, up from 5 percent in 1964. Less than 30 percent of all kids in high school take daily gym classes. An obese teenager runs a 75 percent risk of being an obese adult.

More than 55 percent of all American adults are overweight—is it any wonder that our kids are catching up to us? Obesity in kids is due primarily to two factors—poor eating habits and lack of exercise. Genetics may play a role but, experts say, it accounts for only 50 percent of the total picture. Someone born with a so-called fat gene may never be stick thin, but there's no reason for him or her to be obese.

Obesity is often a family affair. One way or another, it begins in the home, and it can end there, too. Here are my tips on how to raise a happy, well-nourished, healthy child.

BE A GOOD ROLE MODEL. Show me an obese child, and I'll show you a kitchen full of junk food! Your kids are watching you. They eat what you eat. They drink what you drink. If you smoke, they have a greater tendency to do the same. If you don't exercise, they won't exercise.

GOOD BREAKFAST IS ESSENTIAL. Studies have shown that kids who eat 15 grams (half ounce) of protein in the morning do better in school and in sports. Involve your kids in the preparation. Let them scramble eggs, cook some uncured sausage, or Boca links (they're all soy and my favorite), or heat up some cereal. No time? No problem! Throw some soy milk and fruit in the blender with a scoop of protein powder. For extra calcium, add a few tablespoons of dried milk. You've got a great breakfast in thirty seconds.

BROWN BAG THEIR LUNCH. Stuff their lunch bags with healthy but tasty stuff. Good choices are natural peanut butter or fresh turkey on whole-grain bread, pasta salad, fruits and veggies with dip. A small dessert is fine as long as the rest of the meal is basically sound. Get involved in their school lunch program. Get rid of the vending machines selling soda and candy. Make sure the school has a salad bar and offers students other healthy options.

ENCOURAGE SPORTS. Get your kids moving—it's the best way to keep them at normal weight. Kids are loaded with energy—they need to burn it off. All kids should be involved in some sports activity, such as soccer, baseball, hockey, football, swimming, track, or cross-country running.

GIVE THEM PRAISE. I may not have a Ph.D. in psychology, but I did raise two kids. I know that kids can be exasperating at times, but it's a big mistake to constantly criticize. Give them encouragement.

Offer constructive criticism. Give as much love as you can. Happy kids will be less likely to need Prozac or Ritalin.

FIND A NUTRITIONALLY ORIENTED HEALTH-CARE PRACTITIONER. Take your children to a pediatrician who doesn't stress antibiotics, Ritalin or Prozac, and who is interested in their diet and lifestyle, not just their medical problems. If a child has difficulty making the right food choices, get him or her a consultation with a qualified registered dietitian—sometimes kids find it easier to listen to someone other than a family member.

GET THEM INTO THE WATER HABIT. Keep your kids away from soda, which loads them up with calories and can deplete them of calcium. Get them into the habit of drinking filtered or bottled water. For flavor, add a twist of lemon, orange, or lime, or buy fruit-flavored water (like Perrier or Poland Spring) that has no calories. Sparkling water like Pellegrino or Gerolsteler also contains minerals, such as calcium.

EXPERIMENT WITH DIFFERENT FOODS. Get out of the meat-chicken-potatoes rut. Give your kids brown rice and vegetables, whole-grain breads and cereals (check out the cereal counter at your natural food store—you'll be surprised by the variety), new vegetables (how about purple potatoes?), and, of course, soy foods.

GIVE THEM A NATURAL COMPLETE VITAMIN/MINERAL. A daily multivitamin/mineral supplement (chewable for small kids) is essential to make sure that your kids are getting all the necessary nutrients they need. It should be free of artificial colors, preservatives, artificial flavors, waxes, or artificial sweeteners, as well as being sugar, wheat, and yeast free.

4

PEAK PERFORMANCE TEENS

About 50 percent of adolescent boys and 25 percent of adolescent girls compete in organized sports programs during the school year. They're the lucky ones! If fitness is a part of your life at an early age, it's likely to become a lifelong habit. Teen athletes have a head start on maintaining a lifetime of good health.

As great as exercise is for the body and the mind, however, it can put extra stress on a growing body. To achieve maximum benefit from their workout, physically active teens need to take special care of their bodies. Adolescents are particularly vulnerable to poor nutrition and haphazard training habits. Oftentimes, overzealous coaches can contribute to the problem. Neglecting to eat well, train sensibly, and get enough rest will not only affect a teen's ability to perform well in his or her sport and in school, but could lead to unnecessary injury. It's essential for teen athletes to be armed with the information they need so that they stay on top of their game without endangering their health. As a father of two grown children, I know that kids have minds of their own. I also know that teenagers today are smart and, if they understand why something is important, they are more likely to do it. Therefore, I have written this chapter for both teen athletes and parents. I hope that you both can work together to create an environment that is conducive to success on and off the playing field.

Eat to Win

Good nutrition is the foundation for successful athletic performance. It provides the fuel for succeeding in sport and in the classroom, as well as the energy to pursue a social life. I recommend that all teens review the chapter on Peak Performance Nutrition, because the basic rules of eating well are the same. There are some important differences, however, between adults and teens. Unlike an adult, a teenager's body is still developing and growing. Teenage athletes burn up an enormous number of calories. First, they're extraordinarily active. Second, they have more muscle mass than adults, and muscle burns more calories than flab. Third, they need energy to keep growing. Active kids need to eat three meals a day and several healthy snacks. In my opinion, any coach who puts a teenager on a low-calorie diet that leaves the him or her hungry has no business working with kids! Of course, it's fine to teach kids how to eliminate junk food and make healthy food choices, but it's not right to starve them. If a teen is eating correctly, he or she should be able to maintain the right weight. If a teen cannot achieve a weight goal set by a coach without resorting to starvation (or, as I'll discuss later, drugs), then he or she needs to pick another sport that is more suited to his or her body. Here are some tips you need to eat to win.

THREE SQUARES A DAY AND SNACKS. An active, developing body needs to eat three meals a day and two to three snacks. That means not skipping breakfast or missing lunch, two key meals meant to get you through the day.

KIDS NEED CARBS. Forget about high-protein diets! Carbs provide the primary source of energy for teen athletes—about 65 percent of a teen's daily calories should be in the form of carbs. Of course, not all carbs are created equal. Whole grain bread is a carb, but so are french fries and soda! Best choices are unrefined, whole-grain carbs that have not been depleted of their fiber or nutrients. By the way, like adults, teens need fiber! Fiber makes you feel full, and prevents you from getting hunger pangs too soon after eating. Carbs work best when combined with some protein. For example, an ideal breakfast would include a healthy cereal (Arrowhead Mills miniwheats are great) with either soy milk or low-fat cow's milk. Sprinkle some sunflower seeds on top for added protein and some good fat (which helps you feel satisfied). On days that you are training before school, however, you may want to eat lighter. Another great choice is a healthy breakfast shake (Juice Plus or Spiruteen are good choices) made with fresh fruit and a table spoon of flaxseed oil. (Flaxseed oil is a rich source of good fat.) You can mix these shakes with cow's milk, but real milk may be too heavy before working out. Rice Dream or fat-reduced soy milk may be a better choice on those mornings. Add ice to make a thicker shake. Be sure to pack a snack to refuel your cells after your workout—never leave home without one!

LEAN PROTEIN IS BEST. Teens need protein, but not in massive quantities. (The right amount of protein grams per day should equal body weight in pounds multiplied by .6–.9 percent. A teen weighing about 110 pounds needs anywhere from 66 to 99 grams of protein daily.) Heavy, fatty protein choices will weigh you down. Stick to lean cuts of meat, chicken breast, and fish.

SNACKING. Teens need to have access to healthy snacks at home and on the run. At home, keep fresh, washed fruit in the refrigerator. Kids love grapes (make it really easy, take them off the stem), pineapple chunks, melon balls—anything that they can easily grab. Fruit has no protein, so it should be combined with a small bit of protein, like a handful of nuts. Fresh vegetables and a yogurt-based dip is another great snack for active teens. Sliced apples with natural peanut butter is also a popular and easy-to-make snack.

Teens should never leave the house without a snack in their backpack or purse. Hungry kids will grab for anything in sight, including high-fat, low-nutrient foods from fast-food restaurants. Remember, kids don't want to carry ice packs with them, so be sure to pack foods that won't perish. Nuts and dried fruit is a good choice for a portable snack, as is a peanut butter and jelly sandwich on whole-grain bread. A high-carb sports drink (designed for preworkout) or a high-quality sports bar is okay, too, but be sure that it is not a candy bar in disguise.

DON'T SKIP LUNCH. For teens, lunch is every bit as important as breakfast. By midmorning, many teens begin to feel groggy, especially if they've been sitting in a classroom. Lunch is the meal that recharges body and mind. A can of soda and a bag of chips is not lunch—it's a junk-food feast. It may provide an immediate lift, but a crash will follow rapidly, and lead to poor performance for the rest of the day. If possible, bring lunch from home. Good choices are a lean roast-beef sandwich or turkey on whole-grain bread with lettuce and tomato, or pasta salad (preferably made with DeBoles pasta, a combination of artichoke flour and semolina wheat—it's higher in nutrients and fiber than regular pasta). If teens buy lunch at school, they should avoid the junk selections. Many high schools today have salad bars, and healthier choices than in the past. An occasional slice of pizza is fine for lunch (not every day—it's a bit high in saturated fat).

FAST FOOD. Fast-food restaurants can be treacherous for teens, but even there, they can make the right food selections. Many fast-food restaurants offer a grilled chicken salad or sandwich, a much better choice than cheeseburgers and fries. Skip the soda! Drink water, seltzer, or fruit juice. Teens should avoid caffeinated beverages—if a pick-me-up is needed, in the afternoon, they are not eating right or getting enough rest.

DINNER. Teens should not eat too late or too much—digestion is hard work and a big meal can keep them up at night. Dinner should be filling, but not heavy. Pasta, salad, soup, grilled fish, and chicken are good choices. A fresh fruit sorbet or yogurt and fruit and honey are good desserts.

STAY HYDRATED. Teens may have more problems regulating body temperature than adults (they're metabolically more active, therefore, they generate more heat). Teens need to drink lots of fluid before, during, and after exercise. Sports drinks are particularly appealing to this age group.

TAKE YOUR ANTIOXIDANTS. Teenage athletes need to take antioxidant supplements to help repair the oxidative damage to their muscles caused by intense exercise. Brightly colored fruits and veggies are also a great source of natural antioxidants.

TEENAGE GIRLS HAVE SPECIAL NEEDS. Teenage girls should get at least 1200 mg. calcium daily, but more than half do not get even 50 percent of that amount. Low calcium intake during the years of peak bone growth can lead to osteoporosis. Iron is another mineral that teenage girls need, but may not get in sufficient quantity. Parents should keep an eye out for signs of iron-deficient anemia, the primary one being excess fatigue.

Lifestyle Tips

TEENS NEED SLEEP. Teenagers are chronically sleep deprived, especially those who wake up early to train before school. Kids need sleep—hormones associated with growth and development are secreted at night at a higher level than during periods of wakefulness. Experts now believe that teens need more sleep than adults, yet many get less. Teen athletes often work late into the night to finish homework. It's particularly important for parents to teach kids time-management techniques that can help prevent them from feeling overwhelmed. In addition, weekends should not be filled with activities every second. Teens need time to catch up on their sleep (and to catch their breath).

BEWARE OF CRAZY COACHES. Overtraining is a major problem with teen athletes. Some coaches push kids beyond their limits, which is harmful both physically and emotionally. If a teen is getting injured frequently, or has to take painkillers constantly, it's a sign of overtraining or poor training. A teen athlete should feel free to say, "Hey, my (knee, shoulder, leg) hurts today, I can't play." No teen should be subjected to a coach who is verbally abusive, or constantly tearing him down.

ALCOHOL. Wine, beer, and sugary coolers that are shamelessly marketed to kids are an unnecessary source of sugar and calories. If you're trying to stay sleek and strong, alcohol is your worst enemy.

HAVE FUN. So many kids today are overprogrammed and overstressed! Teens need time for fun. No teen athlete should be so busy with school and training that he or she doesn't have time to hang out with friends, go to a party on the weekends, shop at the mall, catch up on email, or simply sit and read a good book!

Avoiding the Anabolic Steroid Trap

Teenage athletes are at particular risk of abusing anabolic steroids. Adolescents are forever looking for a quick fix—they are impatient by nature and want to see immediate results. Many feel if they can get bigger, stronger, and faster by taking a pill, why not? In order for kids to understand why they shouldn't be messing around with steroids, they need to know the facts.

Anabolic steroids are basically synthetic versions of testosterone. Testosterone builds tissue and masculinizes the body. As boys enter puberty, testosterone levels soar—it's the hormone that builds muscle, stimulates the growth of reproductive organs, is responsible for sex drive, and enhances energy. Girls and women have testosterone, too, but males have much higher levels of testosterone.

Anabolic steroids were developed to treat low levels of testosterone in men. Athletes began using them in the 1960s and 1970s to enhance performance but, in 1988, Congress passed the Anti-Drug Abuse Act, making the distribution or possession of anabolic steroids illegal, unless prescribed by a physician for a recognized medical condition. In 1990, Congress passed an even tougher law making anabolic steroids a controlled substance, increasing the penalties for possession or selling these products. All competitive sports organizations have banned the use of anabolic steroids. Despite the tough laws, there is a thriving black market in steroids. A recent survey of high-school seniors revealed that 3 to 5 percent of males and .5 percent of females had at one time used anabolic steroids.

The use of anabolic steroids by teenagers is particularly dangerous, because these powerful drugs can cause serious and long-term side effects. One problem is that teenagers tend to take megadoses of steroids—they think that if a little works, a lot will work even better. There is a delicate balance of hormones in the human body. Taking too much of one can easily throw off that balance and have a destructive effect.

I'm not saying that anabolic steroids won't grow muscle—they do, but at a great cost. Some studies suggest that they are addictive, and that users show the same signs of denial and abuse as drug addicts. Here are some of the other untoward side effects:

TEENAGE BOYS

Premature skeletal maturation, which could stunt growth
Reduced sperm count, shrunken testicles
Development of breasts
Increase in bad cholesterol, which could lead to heart disease
Increased aggression and hostility
Dampening of the immune system

TEENAGE GIRLS

Premature skeletal maturation, which could stunt growth
Growth of facial hair
Deepening voice
Anger, aggression
Increase in bad cholesterol

The effects of steroids are not permanent; you lose the gains shortly after discontinuing the drugs. Because these drugs are obtained, and are often imported from countries outside the United States, the FDA does not monitor their quality. The product may be tainted, which increases the risk.

A testosterone gel is shortly coming to market in the United States for older men with flagging testosterone levels, and it's getting a great deal of media attention. Teenagers may view this discussion about testosterone as a sign of a growing acceptance of testosterone in general and anabolic steroids, in particular, by the medical community. Nothing could be further from the truth! Testosterone replacement in men is still very controversial and not without significant side effects. In fact, men who take testosterone are closely monitored by their physicians. There is one big difference between testosterone gel users and teens who use anabolic steroids. The teenage body is still growing and developing, and more likely to suffer the consequences of hormonal imbalance, whereas an older body is not.

What about the so-called T-boosters (andros) for kids? They're weaker than the real stuff, but can also cause similar side effects. So, in my opinion, they provide the *worst* of both worlds.

Beware of Diet Pills

Many teens use diet pills that contain high doses of stimulants (like ephedrine, dexedrine, and caffeine). Although these pills are sold over the counter, they can cause real problems if they are abused. Teens tend to ignore dose recommendations and take more than they should. In the wrong body, stimulants can trigger hidden heart problems that can be lethal. Even if used correctly, these products can cause jumpiness and jitteriness. Another problem is that their effects are short-lived, leading to a surge of energy, then a crash, and a need to take another pill. My advice—steer clear of these products.

Safer Options for Teenagers

In general, I feel that all it takes to get a teenage body stronger is good nutrition, smart and consistent training, and enough rest. A multivitamin with antioxidants can help fill in the nutritional gaps. In the competitive world of high-school athletics, many teenagers feel they need something extra to give them an edge over the other players. Fortunately, there are better options than anabolic steroids. Here is my short list of hormone-free natural supplements that are reasonably safe, but still may build muscle and enhance performance without wreaking havoc on the body.

CREATINE. Chances are, if you're a teenage athlete, you already know about creatine or are taking it yourself. Creatine is essential for the production of *ATP*, the fuel that runs the body. It forces muscle cells to retain fluid, giving them a pumped look. Some studies suggest it can enhance performance and endurance. Because it adds bulk (which could slow you down), creatine is more for strength athletes, weight lifters, and football players than long-distance runners. The plus side of creatine is that it is being used by hundreds of thousands of people with virtually no side effects. (In rare instances, I've heard, it's caused muscle cramps.) The negative side is that it's only been used for a few years, and the long-term effects are unknown. However, as sports supplements go, it's probably the best researched and the most widely used. Start with a loading dose of 20–25 grams per day for five days. (Take 5–6 grams of creatine up to four times daily with a meal or snack.) After five days, take 2 grams daily (1 gram at breakfast and 1 at lunch). Creatine works best when combined with carbohydrate.

RIBOSE. Ribose is a simple sugar found in all living cells. Your body produces ribose on its own—it is essential for the formation of ATP, which you need for energy. Studies have shown that ribose supplements can increase ATP production. Ribose may be particularly helpful for high-school athletes who often train every day, depleting their ATP stores and not giving their bodies enough time to bounce back. Take 3–5 grams per day. Take half your dose an hour before exercise and half immediately following exercise. If you want to take it only once a day, take it after exercise.

WHEY PROTEIN. Whey protein is derived from milk products. It is a rich source of amino acids, including the branched-chain amino acids needed to repair muscle. Whey protein is highly absorbable by the body. Having adequate amounts of protein on hand is necessary to maintain muscle growth and prevent muscle breakdown. (People who are allergic to milk or are lactose intolerant should avoid whey products.) Mix two tablespoons whey protein powder in liquid daily.

For more detailed information on the supplements listed here, check the Hot Hundred.

5

PEAK PERFORMANCE SEX

The same tools that help you perform your best in the gym, on the playing field, and at work will help you lead an active and vibrant sex life. The flip side is that the same downers that sap you of energy and wreak havoc on your body can help destroy your sex life. In order to stay svelte, sexy, and in the game, you need to maintain a supportive life style.

Sexual problems are quite common from midlife on, in both men and women. About 25 percent of men over fifty have experienced *erectile dysfunction* (ED), the inability to achieve or maintain an erection sufficient to sustain intercourse. Although women have not been studied as much as men, there is a growing body of evidence that menopause can interfere with libido and sexual function.

The introduction of Viagra in 1998 with great hype and fanfare has led many people to believe that a pill can solve all sexual problems. Not so! Viagra works for many men, but not all. Remember, Viagra is a performance pill, but it doesn't make you want to perform. That is, it has no effect on loss of libido, a major cause of sexual problems in men and women. In addition, Viagra can be downright dangerous for men with heart conditions (a common cause of ED), and has resulted in more than five hundred deaths, not to mention other untoward side effects, such as headaches and blackouts. And it doesn't seem to work for women. Personally, I feel that Viagra should be treated as a last resort for ED, not the first line of treatment. It needs to be used with great caution. My advice is to try simple, natural things that do not produce a myriad of potentially dangerous side effects first.

Many of the problems that can dampen your sex life are entirely avoidable. They are due to poor health habits which, over years, damage every vital system within the body. When it comes to sexual function, the best medicine is prevention. Taking care of yourself from your teen years on can make a tremendous difference in your sex life in the following decades. Even if you have already shown signs of slowing down, it's not too late to do something about it. (Supplements mentioned below that are also included in the Hot Hundred are designated by an asterisk.)

YOUR HEART AND YOUR SEX LIFE. About half of all cases of ED are caused by *atherosclerosis*, the clogging of the arteries delivering blood to the heart and other vital organs. Maintaining normal cholesterol levels (under 200 mg/dl) is one way to protect your heart. It's very important to keep your levels of HDL, or good, cholesterol high. Studies have linked lower HDL to a greater risk of ED. The health of your heart is directly connected to your diet. Watch what you eat! A diet high in saturated fat (from meat and dairy products) can increase the risk of heart disease. (For more information on food, turn to the chapter Peak Performance Nutrition.)

YOUR WEIGHT AND YOUR SEX LIFE. Obesity, especially in men, can interfere with sexual function. Why? Obesity is often linked to other physical problems, such as heart disease and diabetes, which can cause sexual problems. Given the fact that 25 percent of all American adults are obese, we are looking at an epidemic of male sexual dysfunction. Obesity can affect a woman's sex life too. Women who feel that they are unattractive are often reluctant to engage in any activity that involves taking off their clothes!

CIGARETTES ARE KILLING YOUR SEX LIFE! Studies have shown that cigarette smokers are twice as likely to suffer from ED than nonsmokers. Why? Cigarette smoking is a leading cause of atherosclerosis, which reduces the flow of blood throughout the body, including the penis. In all likelihood, smoking can also hamper a woman's ability to become aroused and enjoy sex for the same reason—you need adequate blood flow to the pelvis area for normal sexual function. Ninety percent of heavy smokers will suffer damage to the penile artery.

MIND YOUR HORMONES. Changing hormone levels from midlife on in both men and women can affect sexual desire and function. About 30 percent of all men past midlife will experience a dip in testosterone levels that could affect sex drive. Women also experience a dramatic drop in estrogen, progesterone, and testosterone that can also hamper libido and function. Hormone-replacement therapy is becoming popular for both men and women; however, it is not without some risk. Sex hormones (estrogen and testosterone) can stimulate the growth of hormone-sensitive cancers; therefore, I view them as a last resort. Several of the supplements that I recommend in this book can also boost hormone levels, such as DHEA* and T-Boosters*. However, if you take any kind of hormone, natural or otherwise, please do so under a doctor's supervision.

ALCOHOL IS A DOWNER. Although alcohol lowers inhibitions, it can actually hurt your sex life. More than two alcoholic drinks daily can decrease sex drive and lower testosterone levels. Need I say more?

STRESS AND SEX DON'T MIX. Stress hormones can shut down the production of sex hormones, which is very unsexy. Ironically, many prescription antidepressants and anti-anxiety drugs can interfere with sexual function. So, try natural remedies first. If you're stressed out, try to reduce exposure to stressful people and situations. Give yourself a time each day when you turn on the answering machine, turn on some music, put up your feet and relax! Try aromatherapy. The scent of lavender is soothing, and there are absolutely no side effects. Even a twenty-minute stress break can be a lifesaver if you use it to decompress. Supplements such as arctic root* or phosphatidylserine* can help control stress hormones. *Kava* is a herb from the South Pacific that is great for relieving anxiety and putting you in a good mood. Take one to two capsules before bedtime. Recognize that stress should be taken seriously, and that you need to make time for yourself.

EXERCISE IS AN APHRODISIAC. People who exercise have more sex than people who don't. A recent study of more than eight thousand women between the ages of eighteen and fifty found that those who did aerobic exercise at least three times per week reported better sex lives than sedentary women. Studies of men have yielded similar results. There are several reasons why exercise makes you sexier. Clearly, exercise does wonders for your body and your mind. It boosts levels of *endorphins*, happy hormones in your brain that elevate mood and create a sense of well being, which is conducive to sex. Second, exercise improves blood flow, which is important for arousal. Third, it helps prevent the physical problems (like clogged arteries) that can wreck your sex life. And, finally, exercise makes you look better and gives you more body confidence, which is also important.

KEEP YOUR PROSTATE HEALTHY. The prostate is a small, walnut-shaped gland that surrounds the part of the urethra that is located under the bladder. Enlarged prostate, or BPH (benign prostate hypertrophy) is very common in men over forty. It won't make you impotent and it doesn't cause cancer, but it is uncomfortable and can make sex uncomfortable. BPH is caused by an increase in a more potent form of testosterone, dihydrotestosterone (DHT) which occurs during middle age. This bad testosterone not only irritates the prostate, but can make you bald! My advice is—don't let it get the better of you! Keep your prostate healthy. I recommend that all men over forty take the herb *saw palmetto*, which helps protect against potent forms of testosterone that can irritate the prostate. Take 160 mg. saw palmetto daily, or a prostate-specific formula. I take a combination of saw palmetto, pygeum, nettles, beta sitosterol*, zinc*, and lycopene twice daily.

In addition, be sure that you're getting enough *zinc*, a mineral that enhances the health of the male reproductive system. There is a higher concentration of zinc in the male prostate than anywhere else in the body. No wonder zinc-rich foods, such as oysters, have earned reputations as aphrodisiacs. Low levels of zinc have been linked to low sperm count. Make sure you are getting at least 30 mg. zinc daily.

Soy-based foods (tofu, miso, tempeh, soy milk) are a great source of natural hormones that appear to protect the prostate from DHT. If you don't eat these foods routinely, drink a soy milk shake daily—it's the easiest way to be sure to get enough soy.

OVERCOMING THE MENOPAUSE HURDLE. The sudden hormonal shifts that occur in midlife women can cause many unpleasant side effects that interfere with sex. Hot flashes, vaginal dryness, and insomnia don't exactly make you feel amorous. These problems can be overcome easily and naturally. Soy products (tofu, soy milk, soy cereals, soy beans) contain plant estrogens that can help relieve menopausal symptoms. They also appear to be protective against cancer. (However, women with prexisting breast cancer or other hormone-sensitive cancers should only use these products under the guidance of their physicians.) A cup of soy milk, or two ounces of tofu daily, could make a big difference in how you feel.

Black cohosh is a wonderful herb for helping to soothe menopausal symptoms. Studies conducted in Europe have shown that it is both effective and safe for short-term use, and can relieve insomnia, mild depression, hot flashes, and so on. Take 40 mg. daily for up to six months. (There have not been any long-term studies; however, this herb has been used for hundreds of years with no history of problems.)

If these simple, natural solutions don't work, you may need to use hormone-replacement therapy, at least for a while. Ask your doctor about natural estrogen and natural progesterone. Although these hormones are synthetically produced, they are identical in structure to the hormones produced by a woman's body, unlike the commercial brands of hormones most often prescribed to women. Many women find that natural hormones do the job as well or even better than synthetic hormones, with fewer side effects. A recent study suggests that natural progesterone is better for the heart than the synthetic progesterone most commonly prescribed to women. Since natural hormones are not marketed as aggressively by drug companies, your doctor may not tell you about them. It's up to you to ask!

Several other supplements that I recommend for enhancing libido and improving sexual function are discussed in the following sections.

ARGININE*. *Arginine* is an amino acid that can increase the body's production of nitric oxide, a gas which is needed to open blood vessels, which in turn improves blood flow to the penis. Theoretically, the better the blood flow, the easier it is to achieve and maintain an erection. Arginine is one of the most popular natural sexual-enhancement supplements on the market. Used alone or in combination with other herbs, arginine seems to get good results. I've spoken to scores of happy users who feel that arginine has made a huge difference in their ability to enjoy sex. Take 1500 mg. twice daily of time-released arginine. Keep in mind that arginine doesn't work for everybody, and there are some conditions that may require medication or other treatments.

CORDYCEPS*. *Coryceps* is a rare Chinese mushroom that, for centuries, has been used as a tonic to improve athletic performance and sexual function. It may increase blood flow to the pelvic region, which would improve the ability to achieve and maintain an erection in men, as well as sexual function in women. Look for a new herbal product containing cordyceps, ginkgo and L-arginine. It's a winning combination! Take two 525 mg. capsules daily.

DAMIANA. This herb is a traditional treatment for depression and male sexual problems in Central America and Mexico. Interestingly, no one knows how or if this herb works—scientists have been unable to detect any physiological activity. Of course, that doesn't mean that it doesn't work, only that we don't know much about damiana. Due to its centuries' old reputation as an aphrodisiac, it is often included in sex-enhancing herbal formulas. In very high doses, it may induce a mild euphoria which has been compared to marijuana—the downside is, in high doses, it could also give you a nasty case of diarrhea! The usual dose for damiana is 400–1200 mg. daily.

DHEA*. *DHEA* is a steroid hormone found in the human body. Similar to other sex hormones, levels of DHEA decline with age. Two separate studies have shown that DHEA supplements can enhance sex drive and performance in both men and women. In one study, women who were given DHEA for four months reported a sharp increase in sex drive. In another study of twenty men, DHEA not only increased their libido, but improved erectile function, orgasm, and overall satisfaction with their sex lives. There's the catch: Like other hormones, DHEA should only be supplemented if the body is not making enough on its own. Therefore, you need to have your DHEA levels checked by your doctor before taking it. DHEA levels should be monitored by a physician to be sure that you are taking the right amount. Women, in particular, need to be careful with DHEA. It could produce a boost of testosterone which can cause some unpleasant side effects like facial hair and deepening of the voice. The usual dose is 25 mg. daily for women, 50 mg. for men, taken first thing in the morning. DHEA is not for anyone under forty. If you're forty or over, have your DHEA level checked with a simple saliva test by a nutritionally oriented physician.

GINKGO*. Well known as the herb for your brain, ginkgo is fast becoming famous as the herb for better sex. Several studies confirm that ginkgo can enhance sexual function in both men and women. In fact, in one study published in the *Journal of Urology*, ginkgo improved erectile function in men with a history of sexual problems. Ginkgo works by preventing blood platelets from clumping, thereby improving circulation throughout the body. Take up to two 60 mg. capsules daily.

HORNY GOAT WEED*. Often called *herbal Viagra*, horny goat weed has been used for hundreds of years in China to treat male sexual dysfunction. It is purported to enhance libido, strengthen erections, and improve stamina. A word of caution: Some herbalists believe that horny goat weed is so similar in action to Viagra that, like Viagra, it should not be used by people taking nitroglycerin for heart conditions. Take three 1000 mg. capsules daily.

MACA*. This Peruvian herb is being touted as an aphrodisiac and performance enhancer for both men and women. Maca has traditionally been used to treat menopausal symptoms in women, as well as sexual dysfunction in men. What makes this herb so versatile? It contains *sterols*, the building blocks of sex hormones, critical for sexual desire and function for men and women. Recent animal studies suggest that maca maybe useful as a treatment for erectile dysfunction (impotence). It also boosts energy, which helps improve stamina both in and out of the bedroom. There are no known side effects, which makes maca safer than some of the prescription treatments for erectile problems. Take three 525 mg. capsules daily.

MUIRA PUAMA. Known as *potency wood*, this Brazilian herb is reputed to enhance libido and improve sexual function in men and women. According to one French study of 262 men with sexual problems, this herb can rev up your sex drive and improve erectile function.

The usual dose is 750–1500 mg. up to three times daily. There are no known side effects but, at high doses, a small percentage of men reported upset stomach and headaches.

PHEROMONES*. *Pheromones* are substances secreted by animals (and humans) that are believed to affect reproductive behavior. Although you can't actually smell pheromones like other scents and odors, we sense them through the vomernasal organ located in the nasal cavity. Pheromones are a form of nonverbal communication: They send out a message to potential partners that we are ready, willing, and interested. Recently, several brands of synthetic pheromones have been brought to market. A few well-done studies show that they appear to make you more attractive to the opposite sex. So, if you have romance on your mind, dab some pheromones on your neck and wrist, and see what happens. . . .

TRIBULUS*. Tribulus has long been used as a treatment for depression and sexual problems. The herb contains steroidallike compounds, such as saponins, which could increase libido. Some studies suggest that tribulus raises levels of LH (luteinizing hormone), which should increase testosterone production in men; therefore, it should not be used by men with prostate problems. Tribulus is often used in formulas for male potency. Take two 125 mg. tablets daily.

VELVET DEER ANTLER*. Velvet deer antler is the soft outside covering on the young antler, discarded by the animal each year when he matures. For centuries, velvet deer antler has been highly prized as a traditional medicine, and especially for its purported sexual-enhancing properties. Recent studies suggest that velvet deer antler may boost testosterone levels in men, which could increase libido and energy. Take one 70 mg. capsule daily.

YOHIMBE*. Yohimbe, extracted from a bark of a tree native to west Africa, has been used as a traditional treatment for sexual dysfunction and loss of libido. A stronger version of yohimbe (yohimbine hydrochloride) is sold as a prescription drug. Yohimbe dilates blood vessels, improving blood flow to the penis. It works well for some people, but there is the risk of dangerous side effects in high doses. Yohimbine HCL (the prescription drug) can cause a rapid drop in blood pressure, dizziness, and anxiety. Although the weaker yohimbe herb is reputedly safer, there is the same potential for problems. Therefore, I prefer to err on the side of caution. If you use yohimbe, do so under the supervision of a physician. I would try safer things first, such as maca, gingko, and horny goat weed. Take one 500 mg. capsule up to three times daily.

6

PEAK PERFORMANCE TIPS FOR YOUR BRAIN

It takes more than sheer muscle to be a winner—you also need to keep your brain pumped and ready for action. Good concentration and focus are important for optimal physical and mental function. A fuzzy, tired brain can keep you from achieving your goals at work, school, or at play.

As you know, I'm a great believer in the use of supplements, when appropriate, as a tool to enhance health and prevent disease, but I also know their limitations. When it comes to preserving and enhancing your brain power, lifestyle and nutrition are even more important than relying on pills, potions, or so-called smart drugs. Of course, the right supplements can help keep you sharp, smart, and well focused, but they can't do the job alone. So, first things first! Before I talk about supplements, I'd like to review some basic things you can do that will keep your brain in peak performance mode.

Get Enough Sleep

It doesn't get any simpler than this! Get in your bed, turn out the lights, and let yourself sleep seven to nine hours per night, depending on your particular needs. If you don't wake up feeling refreshed, or if you tire easily during the day, it's a sign that you need more sleep. If you do, you're not alone: Most Americans don't get enough sleep, and are suffering the effects of sleep deficiency. A lack of sleep will result in poor concentration, irritability, and even depression. Clearly, you can't perform at your best if you are exhausted.

There are two kinds of sleep: *rapid eye movement sleep* (REM) and non-REM. Each night, we experience four to six sleep cycles, each consisting of REM and non-REM sleep. There are two types of non-REM sleep: stage 2 and the much deeper form, called *delta sleep*. Delta sleep is critical for your body. It is during this time that the largest spurt of growth hormone is released during a twenty-four hour period. It is a time of cell growth, repair, and recovery. REM sleep appears to be more involved in mood and mental function. Studies have shown that people who don't get enough REM sleep have difficulty focusing or thinking clearly in the morning. In fact, when people are chronically deprived of REM sleep, they are likely to become confused, agitated, and have memory problems.

People who have difficulty falling asleep and/or staying asleep often do things inadvertently to sabotage their sleep. Caffeine, alcohol, and cigarettes are stimulants that can disrupt sleep. Obviously, avoid them too close to bedtime. In addition, there are some easy things you can do to improve the quality of your sleep.

STICK TO A ROUTINE. Go to bed at roughly the same every night, and wake up at around the same time every morning.

HAVE A BEDTIME RITUAL. Wind down before bedtime. Read a book (another great way to keep your brain fit). Listen to soothing music. Light a scented candle (lavender is soothing) and let your body know that it's time to rest.

NO LATE DINNERS. Don't eat too close to bedtime. Give your body at least two hours to digest dinner before going to sleep. Avoid taxing your digestive system with heavy meals at night.

SAY NO TO SLEEPING PILLS. Sleeping pills induce a chemical sleep that can leave you groggy and tired. They can also be addictive, meaning that the doses often have to be increased to maintain the same effectiveness. My advice is to pass on them, and try gentler, natural remedies. Several herbal sleep aid products contain combinations of chamomile, valerian, and passionflower that can gently induce sleep. Small does of the hormone melatonin can also help reset disrupted sleep cycles. (And I do mean small. For many people, .5–1 mg. does the job! Others may need up to 3 mg. before bedtime to induce sleep.) Only use sleep aids before bed; never take a sleep-inducing drug or supplement before driving.

Feed Your Brain

You know how you have difficulty concentrating when you're hungry? That's because your brain isn't getting the glucose it needs to do its many jobs. The human brain is one of the hardest-working organs in the body, and it requires constant nourishment to fuel its many activities. The wrong kind of food, however, can make your brain even more fatigued. I'm talking about highly sugared, refined carbohydrates (junk food) that make your blood sugar levels soar, then rapidly crash, leaving you depleted, exhausted, and even irritable. Be sure to eat complex carbohydrates with adequate amounts of protein. And never skip meals. Your body and your brain work best when you feed them on schedule.

Remember how your mom used to tell you that fish was brain food? Essential fatty acids found in food, especially fatty fish, are terrific for your brain. The gray matter of your brain is rich in essential fatty acids, which need to be constantly replenished.

Caffeine (in coffee, tea, and chocolate) provides an instant lift, but it wears off soon. So don't rely on endless cups of coffee, tea, or chocolate bars to keep your brain in high gear.

For the long-term health of your brain, don't forget to eat enough antioxidant-rich foods and take antioxidant supplements, like vitamins C, E, and flavonoids. Antioxidants protect your brain from free-radical attack, which can injure healthy brain cells and accelerate aging. Blueberries are a particularly good source of *anthocyanidins*, phytochemicals that animal studies have shown to prevent age-related brain damage.

Exercise Is Great For Your Brain

Many people find that there's a point in the day when they begin to feel tired and can't work as efficiently. They're suffering from brain fog! Some people experience a midmorning slump, for others, it's after lunch or late afternoon. Believe it or not, the best cure for mental fatigue is often exercise. Exercise gets the heart beating faster, which increases the amount of oxygen sent to the brain. Exercise also increases the release of *endorphins*, chemicals that have an opiatelike effect. Endorphins are natural stress relievers and antidepressants. So, when you find yourself nodding off at your desk, take out a pair of running shoes and go out for a brisk walk. If you're at home, take a bike ride or work out to an aerobic tape. You'll feel energized when you're done, and be better able to complete your work. I guarantee that you'll feel more alert and happier.

Exercise Your Brain, Too!

If you don't exercise your muscles, they'll turn to flab. The same is true of your brain. If you don't give it a challenging workout several times a week, it will get weaker. Brain cells communicate with one another via tiny branchlike cells called *dendrites*. When we're young, we have more than enough dendrites to go around but, as we age, it becomes more difficult to make new dendrites. This may be why we find it harder to pick up new skills, like learning a new language or playing an instrument. Yet these are precisely the kinds of activities we need to do to keep growing dendrites. Turn off the television! It's a passive form of entertainment that does not add to your brain power. In order to keep your brain functioning at a more youthful level, you need to challenge it with new activities. Read an intellectually challenging book. Learn how to play bridge. Make it a point to do the crossword puzzle every day. Play word games. Join a book-discussion group. Whatever it is, do something to keep your mind engaged and those neurons working away. I'm not saying that you shouldn't have down time when you can veg out in front of the television, but you also need to schedule enough stimulating activities for your brain.

Avoid Brain Toxins

Many drugs—prescription, over the counter, and illegal—can adversely affect brain function, including memory and alertness. If you are taking a prescription drug, but find that you may not feel as sharp as you like, or are having memory problems, tell your doctor. He or she may be able to prescribe something else. Illegal drugs, like cocaine, amphetamines, and anabolic steroids, can have a damaging impact on brain chemistry. Don't use them!

Watch the Stress

Chronic exposure to stress can accelerate brain aging, interfering with your ability to learn or retain information. *Cortisol*, a hormone released during stress, can injure brain cells, especially in the *hippocampus*, the memory center of the brain. In fact, some researchers believe that chronic exposure to cortisol may be a contributing factor in Alzheimer's disease. Cortisol doesn't just inflict long-term damage; studies have shown that when people are under a great deal of stress they do not learn new tasks as well, or perform at their best. I know that in our harried, modern world, stress is a fact of life, but it doesn't have to be a way of life. Getting enough rest, eating well, getting enough exercise, and learning to cope with stress is critical for your mental and physical well being.

Here, I will recommend some over-the-counter supplements that can also help maintain your brain power. (Supplements that are included in the Hot Hundred are designated by an asterisk.)

For Better Mental Stamina and Concentration

B COMPLEX. When people tell me that they feel that they have difficulty concentrating and are walking around in a funk, the first think I ask them is whether they are getting enough B vitamins. If they're not taking a multivitamin with B complex everyday, they could be lacking enough B-complex vitamins to keep their brains running smoothly and efficiently. B vitamins are important for the production of *ATP*, the fuel that runs the body. Several studies have shown that, when people take B supplements, they're in better moods and think more clearly. Theoretically, B vitamins should be plentiful in the food supply, however, they can be depleted by a high-sugar, high-carbohydrate diet. To fill the gap, take a B-complex supplement daily or look for a multivitamin with B complex. Remember, alcohol drains the body of B vitamins so, during times of mental fatigue or stress, avoid alcohol.

BRAHMI. Also called *gotu kola* and *bacopa*, this Ayurvedic herb is used to boost mental function and concentration. Studies have shown that brahmi can speed up the learning process, enabling test subjects to learn a new task within a shorter period of time than those using a placebo. Brahmi has a mild tranquilizing effect and, historically, has been used as a tonic for the brain. Brahmi can be taken alone, or as part of an Ayurvedic formula designed to enhance brain function. Take up to 3000 mg. daily.

BRANCHED-CHAIN AMINO ACIDS (BCAA)*. Do you find that the longer you exercise, the harder it is for you to stay focused? BCAAs have been shown to give a much-needed mental boost to athletes who frequently overtax their bodies. In fact, studies have shown that BCAAs can help relieve the mental exhaustion that can accompany a vigorous workout, particularly for endurance athletes. BCAAs are three essential amino acids: leucine, isoleucine, and valine which are chemically different from other amino acids, in that they can be easily converted to glucose. So, in addition to building muscle, BCAAs help provide the fuel that energizes both the body and the mind. Take 2–4 grams daily.

NADH*. If you need brain energy, NADH is for you. This co-enzyme has been used to treat chronic fatigue syndrome with some success. Interestingly, it doesn't improve muscle strength, but researchers reported that people who take NADH say they feel more focused and alert. It is also reputed to enhance physical stamina. Since NADH is also an antioxidant, some scientists feel that it may protect against brain aging. Take 2.5–5 mg. daily.

TYROSINE*. There's no substitute for a good night's sleep but, sometimes, work or play keeps you up into the wee hours of the morning. Yet, you're still expected to perform at your peak regardless of your fatigue. Tyrosine could be the supplement to keep you going the day after a late night. Tyrosine is an amino acid that is key to the production of several neurotransmitters, chemical messengers in the brain that help nerve cells communicate with each other. Taken during times of stress, tyrosine can increase energy levels and relieve the symptoms of mental exhaustion. In particular, studies have found that tyrosine helps relieve some of the dip in cognitive function associated with sleep loss. No wonder tyrosine has been studied by the U.S. military as a potential performance enhancer—when you're on the battlefield, you may have little time for sleep but need to stay focused and alert.

Tyrosine, which is also a mood booster, should not be used every day, but only when needed, because it can raise blood pressure. Take 500 mg. twice daily, or up to an hour before working out. Don't take tyrosine late in the day—it could keep you up at night. (Avoid this supplement if you have kidney problems.)

Memory Boosters

PHOSPHATIDYLSERINE*. Known as PS, this supplement is a phospholipid found in cell membranes. PS can both improve memory and boost mental function. The highest concentration of PS is found in the brain. Studies have shown that PS supplements can improve performance of basic mental tasks, such as recalling telephone numbers and names, and memorization. Interestingly, PS appears to help regulate *cortisol*, the stress hormone that has been shown to have a detrimental effect on the brain. PS is a great supplement to take when you're under stress, but still need to think clearly. Take up to 1500 mg. daily.

VINPOCETINE*. Used in Europe for more than twenty years, but new to the United States, this supplement has been shown to help improve blood flow to the brain, which appears to have a positive effect on memory. Vinpocetine also improves the transport of glucose across the blood–brain barrier, making more fuel available to brain cells. In Europe, vinpocetine has been used primarily to treat stroke victims, but is now being explored as a treatment for Alzheimer's disease. Take 10–20 mg. daily.

GINKGO* Gingko biloba is well known for its positive effect on memory and brain function. It is widely prescribed in Europe for age-related memory problems (the serious problems, as well as the run-of-the-mill "where did I leave the keys?" variety). An oft-cited study published in the *Journal of the American Medical Association* found that 120 mg. ginkgo daily for one year improved the mental function of Alzheimer's patients. Some studies conducted in Europe suggest that gingko can also improve cognitive performance in healthy people. Since gingko is also an excellent antioxidant, why not try it? Take up to 120 mg. daily. Some people find that ginkgo can be stimulating, so don't use it too close to bedtime.

HUPERZINE-A. An extract from *club moss*, an herb used in Chinese medicine for centuries, huperzine-A has been shown to improve memory and mental function in patients with Alzheimer's disease. It inhibits *acetylcholinesterase*, the enzyme that breaks down acetylcholine in the brain. Some alternative physicians feel that taking huperzine-A from midlife on may help prevent the type of degenerative changes that lead to senility. Take 50 mcg. daily.

Mood Boosters

SAM-e*. *S-adenosyl-methionine* (SAM-e) is a compound made from amino acid. It has been used in Europe as an antidepressant for close to twenty years, and has recently been brought to the United States as a dietary supplement. Numerous studies support the claim that SAM-e works as well as prescription antidepressants but takes effect faster, and has virtually no side effects. If you feel that you need a mood boost, SAM-e may be the right choice for you. However, depression is a serious problem, so I suggest that you consult with a nutritionally oriented physician before self-medicating. Take up to 800 mg. daily.

DHA*. *Docosahexaneoic acid* is a polyunsaturated omega-3 fatty acid, found in fatty fish, organ meats, and eggs. There are high concentrations of DHA in the gray matter of the human brain. Our modern diet contains very little DHA compared to DHA consumption just one hundred years ago. Low levels of DHA have been linked to depression. According to researchers at the National Institutes of Health, the decline in the consumption of DHA-rich foods may be linked to the rise in the rate of depression in Western countries. There is also some evidence that a deficiency in DHA may contribute to Alzheimer's disease. By the way, in Japan, DHA is touted as a smart drug—it is widely used by students to boost their grades. Take three 250 mg. capsules daily.

7

PEAK PERFORMANCE FOREVER! THE MIDLIFE TUNEUP

If you're reading this chapter, my hunch is you're between the ages of thirty-five and sixty. Regardless of your age or stage of life, the issues are very much the same. You need to keep your body strong to maintain health and vitality. I'm not going to lie to you. As you get older, it's harder to keep your body at peak performance levels, but the good news is that it's not impossible. At any age, you can add muscle, lose fat, and get leaner. You can keep your joints flexible and, in the process, prevent the degenerative diseases that can destroy your lifestyle and rob years from your life. So, let's get started!

There are several peak performance supplements that can help restore stamina and keep you trim and fit. I will discuss them later in this chapter. They are useful tools that can enhance your fitness program, but they are meant to work in synergy with good nutrition and exercise. Before you choose the right supplements for you, you need to understand how to incorporate them into your life to get the results you want.

Goodbye Flab, Hello Muscle

Suffering from middle-age spread? You're not alone. One of life's major challenges is making and keeping muscle. Once you hit your thirties, you begin to lose muscle at a rate of 1 percent per year, or two to four pounds of muscle every decade. By age seventy, we lose as much as 40 percent of our muscle mass. The loss of muscle not only makes you look flabby, but can have a profoundly negative impact on your entire body. When you lose muscle , you get fatter. Muscle is the engine that burns calories. In adults, about one third of energy expenditure is due to muscle. The more muscle you have, the more calories you burn. The less muscle you have, the more those unburned calories are stored as fat. Exercise can help prevent muscle loss and burn excess fat. In fact, a recent study conducted at the University of Colorado showed that female endurance athletes at age fifty-six had the same levels of body fat as normal-weight women of twenty-three. In other words, the fifty-six-year-old athletes were as sleek and trim as women half their age! That's the power of exercise—it is the true rejuvenator.

Maintaining muscle is not just about looking good—it's also critical to your health. Several studies have linked regular exercise with lower rates of *insulin resistance* (a prediabetic condition), heart disease, and cancer. In addition, weight-bearing exercise can help maintain bone mass, which is every bit as important as muscle. As you age, you also lose bone—that's a fact of life. About 24 million Americans also have *osteoporosis*, which literally means *porous bones*. Bones become so thin and brittle that they break easily. By age eighteen, bones reach about 95 percent of their maximum density and, by age thirty-five, both men and women have reached their peak bone mass. After age thirty-five, the body builds less bone to replace the old bone. The older you get, the worse it gets, especially in the first five to ten years after menopause. Men lose bone too, but at a slower rate than women, because they start out with more.

Exercise can slow down bone loss and increase bone mass. Not only that, strong muscles can protect bone and joints from injury. Very simply, if muscles work harder, they can take some of the stress off joints, cartilage, ligaments, and bones. Finally, a man or woman with a well-exercised, fit body is also steadier on his or her feet, which will help prevent injuries down the road. Clearly, muscle can be a true lifesaver.

At any age, it's possible to start rebuilding muscle. Obviously, if you're in your thirties or forties, it's easier to restore muscle, because you haven't lost that much. But studies have shown that even people in their eighties and nineties can rebuild muscle with the right exercise. In fact, studies of nursing home patients in their nineties have shown that just a few weeks of strength training can produce significant increase in muscle strength. Interestingly, researchers have noted that patients who gain strength are more likely to participate in social activities than when they were in a weaker state. To me, this confirms what I have always believed: Exercise can give you a new lease on life.

When it comes to making muscle, the most effective form of exercise is strength training or resistance training (the use of weights and exercise machines) to strengthen specific muscle groups. Muscles grow bigger and stronger when they're forced to work. Activities that involve pushing, pulling, or lifting will increase muscle mass and strength. Aerobic exercise (walking, running, jogging) is great, too. It helps reduce stress, exercises your heart, and improves mood, but it doesn't strengthen all muscle groups equally. A runner can have strong legs but a weak upper body, unless he or she does weight training to enhance upper body strength. I recommend that you try to do a bit of both—strength training and aerobics. Schedule strength training two to three times per week but, on your off days, be sure to do some type of aerobic activity, whether it's walking briskly, cycling, or using a treadmill for thirty minutes. Pressed for time? You don't have to do your exercise all at once—you can break up your aerobic activity into two fifteen-minute or three ten-minute segments and do them at your convenience.

GET HELP. If you've never strength trained before, I recommend that you go to a gym and have a few training sessions with a qualified fitness instructor. It is well worth the money. Exercise machines and weights are an efficient and effective way to build muscle but, if done incorrectly, you can easily be injured. Before picking up a weight or trying a fancy machine, please have an expert show you how to do it correctly! After you know the correct form, you can do it on your own. (If you're over forty or have a chronic medical condition, check with your doctor before embarking on a exercise regimen. He or she may want you to take a stress test to determine the condition of your heart, or may have advice on the best way to exercise.)

WARM UP. Before you lift weights, you need to warm up your muscles to reduce the risk of injury. Walk briskly for five to ten minutes on a treadmill or cycle for five to ten minutes on a stationery bike. This is not a luxury—it's a necessity. Your warmup sends blood and oxygen to muscles throughout the body, prepping them for activity. Cold muscles are more likely to get hurt, and to be sore after your workout.

STRETCH. As part of your warmup, take five minutes to stretch out the muscles in your legs, arms, and back. Simply sit on the floor with your legs extended in front of you. Slowly and gently, bend from the waist and try to touch your toes with your fingertips. Keep your knees straight but soft. *Gentle* is the operative word, don't bounce or force a stretch. Breathe into it gradually. Hold it for ten seconds and stop. Repeat ten times.

GO SLOW. Begin with light weights and do two sets of ten to twelve repetitions for each exercise. Work slowly and carefully. Don't increase your weight until you can do the two sets with relative ease. Don't exercise the same muscle group for two consecutive days: Give your muscles a day or two to recover before exercising them again. Don't overdo it! As any trainer will tell you, the biggest mistake a novice weight trainer can make is doing too much too soon. Older muscles injure more easily than younger muscles. Once you've been injured, there's a good chance that you will turn in your weights and stop exercising, defeating the whole purpose of what you're trying to do.

BREATHE. Breathe in as you get in position to pump—breathe out on exertion. It will give you extra energy!

COOL OFF! End your exercise session with five minutes on the treadmill or exercise bike. It will help speed recovery and reduce post-workout soreness.

Here are some supplements that will help burn fat, increase muscle, and enhance your workout. Supplements that are also included in the Hot Hundred are designated by an asterisk.

ASHWAGANDHA*. Ashwagandha, known as *Indian ginseng*, is a terrific herb for midlife people who need more strength and stamina. In studies of aging animals, ashwagandha has been shown to increase weight and muscle development, and improve memory. Ayurvedic healers boast that ashwagandha is better than ginseng because it increases stamina, but doesn't make you feel edgy. There are other reasons why I like this herb for people who are forty plus. It not only boosts immune function, which declines as we age, but it's also a natural anti-inflammatory, which can relieve joint inflammation and arthritis. Take up to three 4.5 mg tablets daily.

CHROMIUM*. Everyone over forty should be taking chromium! *Chromium*, a trace mineral, is essential for proper glucose and lipid metabolism, and helps the body use insulin more efficiently, which is essential for the preservation and creation of skeletal muscle. Chromium may also help protect against a virtual epidemic among Americans—insulin resistance or Type II diabetes, which can leave you fat, flabby, and vulnerable to heart disease. In *insulin resistance*, the body produces enough insulin, but the cells do not use it efficiently, producing an abnormal rise in blood sugar. Chromium levels decline with age; at the same time, the risk of developing insulin resistance rises exponentially. In fact, 25 percent of all adults over forty will get this condition. Chromium has been studied as an alternative treatment for insulin resistance. According to studies performed by the USDA Human Nutrition Research Center, chromium can lower blood sugar as effectively as prescription medication, but without side effects. A diet high in sugary, processed carbohydrates and fat will increase the likelihood of developing insulin resistance. Many researchers believe that taking chromium, along with a sensible diet, may help prevent it. Most Americans do not get enough chromium from food alone—most fall short of 50 mcg. chromium established as the minimal safe and adequate intake by the National Academy of Sciences. I believe that taking 200 mcg. chromium picolinate (a more absorbable form of chromium) daily is good insurance against insulin resistance.

CONJUGATED LINOLEIC ACID*. CLA is a fatty acid that used to be abundant in red meat and dairy products but, due to modern farming practices, our food supply is now stripped of this fat. Some scientists believe that the loss of CLA in the diet could be directly related to the increase in obesity, and recommend that people take CLA supplements. In fact, recent studies show that CLA can help burn fat and increase lean muscle tissue. CLA will not help you lose weight but, what it may do, is help improve your muscle-to-fat ratio, which will make you appear trimmer. Remember, it's not only what the scale says that counts, it's how you look! A thin person can still look flabby if he or she has poor muscle tone, whereas a person who weighs more can look sleek if he or she has good muscle definition. Several studies have confirmed that CLA is a mild anabolic agent that can help preserve muscle. More good news about CLA: It may help prevent cancer, at least according to animal studies. Similar to omega-3 fatty acids, CLA can lower cholesterol and triglyceride levels and improve insulin sensitivity, which can help reduce the risk of heart disease and diabetes. Take up to three 1200 mg. capsules before meals.

GREEN TEA*. You know that green tea may help prevent cancer, but did you know that it may also help burn fat? Recent studies suggest that green tea contains a unique combination of phytochemicals that can also help you lose weight. In addition to caffeine, which is known to increase *thermogenesis*, the burning of fat, green tea also contains an antioxidant flavonoid called *epigallocatechin* (EGCG), that may hold the key to slimming down. In a twenty-four-hour study designed to measure energy expenditure conducted at the University of Fribourg in Switzerland, researchers gave ten men two capsules of EGCG with each meal. On different days, they gave the men caffeine capsules or a placebo. While taking the green-tea capsules, the men increased overall energy expenditure by 4 percent and fat burning by 10 percent than those taking the caffeine capsules. That amounts to eighty additional calories daily which, over the course of a year adds up to a savings of about 29,000 calories a year or eight and a half pounds. Steep one tea bag in boiling water for two minutes, or take two tablets of extract daily.

HMB*. *B-hydroxy-b-methybutyrate* (HMB) is a metabolite of the branched-chain amino acid leucine that is is naturally produced in the body from foods containing leucine. Several human studies confirm that HMB can increase strength, muscle mass, stamina, and endurance in both men and women. This supplement has become a favorite among young athletes and body builders, but I think it may be perfect for older exercisers who need to hold onto muscle. In one study, thirty-one men and women over seventy participated in a two-day-per-week resistance training for eight weeks. Some were given 3 grams HMB daily, others were given a placebo. After four weeks of training, the HMB increased leg strength over the placebo group. After eight weeks, the HMB group had a greater increase in lean muscle mass, and lost more fat than the placebo group. In a second study of older adults, researchers examined whether resistance training could improve the ability of older people to perform real-life tasks, like the speed in which you can get up from a chair, appropriately called the "Get up and Go Test." Older adults who participated in a resistance training program showed a 2 percent improvement in the "Get up and Go Test," while those who took HMB showed a 7 percent improvement. So, if you're already working out, HMB could be the one supplement that could give you the competitive edge.

HMB is a patented product licensed under several private labels. Take four 1000 mg. capsules daily.

PROANTHOCYANIDINS (PCOs)*. PCOs are a special variety of flavonoids found in the blue, purple, and green pigments of plants (such as blueberries, cranberries, grapes, and pine bark). PCOs are powerful antioxidants that protect against free radicals, which can damage muscle cells and slow down recovery from your workout. In other words, if you don't stop free radicals, these troublesome molecules will wear down your muscles. They also damage every other organ system in the body! In a recent study, PCOs were shown to protect aerobic athletes from free-radical damage and improved endurance. The athletes in the study took 200 mg. pine bark PCOs daily. Interestingly, PCOs not only neutralized free radicals, but actually increased stamina in direct proportion to the degree of suppression of free radicals. Take 150–300 mg. daily.

RHODODENDRON CAUCASICUM*. This hot peak performance supplement is an extract from the *Rhododendron caucasicum* plant that has been used for centuries as a folk medicine in Russia and Asia. It is not only a rich source of antioxidants, but a natural fat blocker. (Please take note—it is not the same as your home-grown rhododendron, which is not safe to eat.) In the Republic of Georgia in Russia, known for its many residents over the age of one hundred, rhododendron is made into a tea that is sipped before meals. This special species of the rhododendron plant is a natural fat blocker—it partially inhibits the action of an enzyme needed for fat absorption, which will help get rid of fat before it is stored in your body. Studies show that rhododendron works especially well with arctic root (European ginseng) to burn fat and promote the formation of lean muscle mass. Take one 50 mg. capsule of rhododendron extract daily before each meal, up to a total of three.

8

PEAK PERFORMANCE TIPS FOR STAMINA AND ENERGY

I'm frequently interviewed on television and radio about issues pertaining to health and fitness. The shows that I enjoy most are those that have call-in questions from listeners. It gives me a chance to see what people are most worried about, and how I can better address their concerns in my books. I have learned that there is one issue that seems to weigh heavily on the minds of people of all ages, in all stages of life, and that is energy, or the lack of it. Believe me, nobody feels that they have enough energy!

The midlife professional complains, "Earl, I would love to exercise, but I'm too tired after work and I have no time during the day."

The young, aspiring high-school athlete laments, "I'm trying to improve my game, but I run out of steam too easily."

The soccer mom admits, "I can barely drag myself out of bed in the morning—just the thought of exercise makes me more tired."

Fatigue may be a universal phenomenon, but not everybody is tired for the same reasons. A high-school student who is perpetually exhausted is tired for different reasons than, for example, his parents or grandparents. In order to solve the energy crises, you need to get to the heart of the problem. First, you need to identify what's making you so tired and, second, you need to get the tools to fix it. Review the following checklist to see if there something in your lifestyle that is sapping you of your precious energy.

(A word of caution: Although most cases of fatigue are due to

225

lifestyle, in some cases, chronic exhaustion can be a sign of a medical problem. If your fatigue isn't helped by making simple changes in your life, be sure to check with your doctor.)

Are You Tired Because . . .

YOU'RE BURNING THE CANDLE AT BOTH ENDS? Do you go, go, go until all hours of the night? Sleep deprivation is a major cause of fatigue, particularly for high-school and college students. Why is sleep so important? Sleep provides you with an opportunity to recharge and reinvigorate every system in your body. If you work hard and play hard, you need your sleep to repair worn cells and make new cells. Americans actually spend 20 percent less time sleeping than they did at the turn of the century. It's not because we're so much busier—back then, without a lot of the more modern conveniences people enjoy today, life was filled with chores and work. The problem is, we have a great many more distractions at night, like television, stores open 24/7, and computers that never rest. If you find yourself dozing at your desk or during class, it's a sign that you need more sleep. Even an extra hour a night could make a huge difference in how you get through the next day.

YOU'RE EATING POORLY? You know who you are! Bagels for breakfast, a pastry for a midmorning snack, a candy bar or a soda in the afternoon as a quick pick-me-up. You're overdosing on refined carbohydrates, foods with little nutritional value. These foods break down rapidly in your bloodstream, providing a steep rise in blood sugar (which makes you feel great) but wears off quickly, leaving you drained and depleted (which make you feel very, very tired). The solution is simple—eat better! Food provides the fuel to keep your body going. In particular, meals containing protein and complex carbohydrates (the slow-burning kind) keep you satisfied longer and provide a steady stream of energy. For breakfast, eat an egg, whole-grain toast, cereal, or a tofu shake with fruit; have fresh fruit and almonds for a midmorning snack, eat lean protein and salad for lunch and dinner. Once you change your eating habits for the better, within a few days, you will feel so good you won't want to stop.

YOU'RE OVERDOING THE CAFFEINE? You're tired, you're looking for a quick fix, so you load up on coffee or cola. You may feel instantly revived but, within an hour or two, you're down again. A cup or two of coffee or tea in the morning is fine, but don't rely on it all the time to restore your energy. It won't work. (And, as you know by now, cola is out of the question!)

YOU'RE JUST OVERDOING IT? I know people who get exhausted just reading over their daily to-do lists. They're so overbooked that there's not a minute to spare. My hunch is that everything on your list is not necessary. Unless the fate of the free world rests on your shoulders, there are things on your list that can wait until tomorrow, or even the next day.

YOU'RE IN A MIDLIFE SLUMP? If you're over forty, and you find yourself saying things like "I can't do what I used to do," or "Where did my energy go?" there are good reasons for how you feel. The fact is that your body may not be making energy as well or as efficiently as it used to. Energy production begins in tiny structures in the cells called *mitochondria*. Mitochondria take material from foodstuffs (glucose, amino acids, and fatty acid), and create the fuel that runs the body. The first part of the process of making energy is called the *Krebs cycle*, which results in the production of ATP, a high-powered fuel. In the second part of the process, *beta oxidation*, ATP is burned to power the building of molecules necessary to run our cells.

When we're younger, our mitochondria churn out more energy than we need but, as we age, things begin to slow down. Our mitochondria begin to show signs of wear and tear. In fact, the same forces that are aging the entire cell (free radicals and exposure to toxins) are causing the mitochondria to age, too. The end result is a subtle, but very real, slowdown in energy production. Without as much energy, cells aren't repaired as rapidly, the body can't function as efficiently, and we begin to feel tired. So what can you do about it? Plenty! Several of the supplements that I recommend help boost the production of ATP (which is good for everybody) but, in particular, help reverse the midlife energy slump. In addition, paying attention to your lifestyle can also make a huge difference in how you feel. If you're body is screaming, "stop pushing so hard," listen to what it is saying. Chances are, you're making things worse by doing all the other things on this check-list—not getting enough sleep, eating on the run, using too much caf-feine, and overbooking yourself.

The following supplements may also help reverse your energy cri-sis. (Supplements that are also listed in the Hot Hundred are desig-nated by an asterisk.)

CARNITINE*. Carnitine is an amino-acidlike substance that is critical for the production of ATP, the fuel that runs the body. The body produces about 25 percent of the carnitine it needs, and gets the rest from food. As we age, levels of carnitine decline, but intense exercise also produces a significant drop in carnitine levels in muscle cells. Therefore, carnitine supplementation is important for young athletes as well as midlife weekend warriors who are running out of steam. Here's what carnitine supplementation may do for you.

Carnitine increases the maximum use of oxygen in athletes, allow-ing them to work out longer without fatigue.

Runners who take two grams of carnitine per day can increase their peak running speed by as much as 6 percent.

Carnitine may help relieve post-workout soreness.

Here's my favorite reason to take carnitine—it's been shown to re-verse the aging process in animals. In a study conducted at the Univer-sity of California at Berkeley, a form of carnitine (acetyl-L-carnitine) was put in the drinking water of twenty-four-month-old rats, the human equivalent of about eighty-five years old. These rats had already begun to show the telltale signs of aging—they were not as active as younger rats and their fur was thinning. Within a month of taking car-nitine, the rats began to show an improvement in energy levels. In fact, according to the researchers, a computer camera that documented the movement of these rats found no difference in the energy level of the carnitine-supplemented rats than that of young rats. Not only that, the carnitine-supplemented rats even looked better! What's even more interesting is that, when the researchers examined the mitochondria of the rats in liver cells, the mitochondria appeared to be rejuvenated, which could explain why the rats had more energy. Whether carnitine can rejuvenate human beings remains to be seen, but I certainly believe that it can improve energy levels. Take two 500 mg. capsules daily of L-carnitine daily.

Co-Q10*. When you turn up energy production in the body, you also produce an unwanted byproduct—free radicals. That's where Co-Q10 comes in. It's a powerful antioxidant, which helps protect cells from free radicals. Not only that, it's also involved in the production of energy within the mitochondria. Co-Q10 is also known as *ubuiquinone* because it is ubiquitous within the body—it is produced by every cell. Similar to carnitine, it also essential for energy production and the two are actually meant to work together. That's why many of the so-called energy formulas on the market include carnitine and Co-Q10. In fact, although some studies have shown that Co-Q10 can improve exercise endurance, I think its effects will be most acutely felt over the long run. I suspect that taking Co-Q10 may help protect against the kind of mitochondrial slowdown that occurs in midlife, and may help reverse it once it happens. Take three 30 mg. capsules daily with meals.

SIBERIAN GINSENG*. There are several different kinds of ginseng (Asian, Korean, American), but Siberian ginseng is the one that is favored most by athletes. Actually, it's not ginseng at all, but a plant that is closely related to the ginseng family. According to numerous Russian studies, Siberian ginseng is a good ergonomic aid. It not only can increase strength and endurance, but helps the body better adapt to environmental stress. This makes it a particularly good supplement for people who exercise in adverse conditions—outdoors in the heat or extreme cold. It also boosts immune function, which makes it a good choice during cold and flu season. Take up to three 400 mg. capsules daily.

NADH*. Energy is what NADH is all about. It's a co-enzyme that stimulates energy production by restoring cellular stores of ATP. In a recent study, NADH supplements were tested on women with chronic fatigue syndrome (CFS), a condition characterized by debilitating fatigue of no known medical origin that lasts for more than six months. (Some researchers believe that CFS is due to the inability of the body to produce enough ATP.) In a study conducted at Georgetown University School of Medicine, researchers gave twenty-six patients 10 mg.

NADH (in the form of Enada, a patented brand) once daily for four weeks. After a four-week break from NADH, the patients were given a placebo. Out of the twenty-six participants, eight felt much better while taking the NADH, as compared to two who felt better on the placebo. Will NADH give healthy people more energy? Try it and see! Take 2.5–5 mg. daily.

RIBOSE*. This is a supplement for people who work out hard, and are serious about their sport. Ribose is simple sugar found in all living cells. It is another ingredient essential for the production of ATP. Although your body produces ribose, during times of extreme exertion you may need more of it, particularly if you engage in strenuous exercise three to four times per week. A small study involving college athletes found that those who took ribose had increased power output and quicker recovery of adenonine nucleotides, the building blocks of ATP, than the placebo takers. In other words, they performed better during their workout and replenished their ATP stores faster after exercise. There are also anecdotal reports from endurance athletes suggesting that ribose does make a difference in both energy levels and recovery time. Ribose is available in capsules, liquid, and powder. Ribose is sold as a single supplement, or in combination with creatine monohydrate. (Some athletes feel that ribose works in synergy with creatine, although this has not been scientifically tested.) The usual recommended dose is three to five grams per day. For best results, divide your dose. Take half your dose an hour before exercise and the second half immediately following exercise.

MAGNESIUM*. Magnesium is essential for the energy-producing cycle within the body. Without it, you can't produce enough energy. Since our bodies don't produce magnesium, we need to get it from foods such as whole grains, nuts, fruits, fish, and legumes. Unfortunately, modern food-processing techniques often strip magnesium from food so, if you eat lots of processed foods, you may be magnesium deficient, which could be hurting your athletic performance. Magnesium supplements may help put you back in the game. Studies suggest that magnesium supplements can enhance physical performance, increase stamina, and even increase lean body mass. Interestingly, magnesium deficiency has been linked to two conditions normally associated with exhaustion: chronic fatigue syndrome and PMS. Try to get more magnesium-rich foods in your life. Take 400 mg. daily. Do not use magnesium if you have kidney problems. Also, stick to my recommended dose; excess magnesium can cause severe diarrhea, particularly in people prone to stomach problems.

9

PEAK PERFORMANCE TIPS FOR RECOVERY

In order to get the most out of each workout session, and be in peak condition for the next, you need to give your body the time and tools it needs to recover properly. Although exercise offers many benefits, vigorous exercise depletes the body of important nutrients. It can also be very stressful on muscles and joints. That's why people feel sore after strenuous physical activity! There are simple things you can do to minimize the downside of exercise, and to fully achieve your fitness goals. First, you need to understand what happens to your body during and after exercise.

PROBLEM: EXERCISE TURNS UP THE HEAT. When you exercise, you need more energy to fuel your increased activity. Your body responds by burning more oxygen to make ATP. On the one hand, this is good. You need the added energy boost. On the other hand, you are also making more free radicals, highly unstable molecules that can be very destructive. Our bodies have their own police force that guard against free radicals—antioxidants, like glutathione, lipoic acid, Co-Q10, and vitamins C and E. However, strenuous exercise can deplete our natural antioxidants, leaving us vulnerable to free radical damage.

SOLUTION: ANTIOXIDANTS. Eating a diet rich in antioxidants, and taking supplemental antioxidants, is one way to give yourself the edge over free radicals.

PROBLEM: YOU USE UP GLYCOGEN. Carbohydrate is stored as glycogen in muscle and liver cells. During a strenuous workout, you will rapidly use up your glycogen stores. *Lactic acid*, a waste product, accumulates in your muscle cells. The end result is tired, sore muscles. The longer you exercise, the worse it can be.

SOLUTION: MORE CARBS. After exercise, you need to restore lost carbohydrate, so that more glycogen can be made. When you eat carbohydrates, your pancreas produces the hormone insulin, which helps transport glucose into the liver and muscle cells (where it is stored as glycogen). Muscle cells are most receptive to insulin immediately following exercise. A light carbohydrate meal, combined with a small amount of protein, right after your workout is the best way to help restore glycogen. (The carbohydrate to protein ratio should be about four to one. Excess protein can actually slow down glycogen recovery.) If you can't get food down after exercise without feeling nauseated, try drinking a high-carbohydrate sports drink designed specifically for recovery. It's best to give yourself a day off after a strenuous workout so that your body has more time to recoup. However, that's not often possible for athletes in training (whether they're pros or on their school team). If you engage in vigorous exercise on consecutive days, you need to be especially careful about your postexercise nutrition. (The rule of thumb for athletes is to consume about nine grams of carbohydrates [thirty-six calories] per 2.2 pounds of body weight everyday.)

PROBLEM: YOU LOSE FLUID. You can lose a surprisingly high amount of body fluid during exercise, especially in warm weather.

SOLUTION: DRINK UP! After your workout, it is very important to restore lost fluid. Water is fine, but some studies suggest that a sports-recovery drink containing electrolytes (sodium, potassium, and magnesium) help replenish fluid more rapidly.

PROBLEM: YOU INJURE MUSCLE. It may surprise you to learn that the way you make muscle is by injuring muscle. When you work your muscles hard, your muscles develop microscopic tears. Your body responds by creating new muscle fibers that are stronger than the old. You know how you can ache after a workout! Some people start hurting immediately after their workout. Others experience a phenomenon called *delayed-onset muscle soreness* (DOMS). The site of injury can become mildly inflamed, causing some swelling and stiffness. It's all normal and actually a good sign—it means that your body has been challenged.

SOLUTION: DON'T OVERDO IT. Although some discomfort goes with the territory, excessive pain is a sign that you are overdoing it in an effort to progress to quickly. It's time to cut back and move more slowly. I don't think that muscle pain is a license to start popping NSAIDs (ibuprofren). These drugs can cause serious side effects, including stomach bleeding and ulcers. If you are so uncomfortable that you can't sleep or sit, try some of the natural solutions. A hot shower after working out followed by an old fashioned muscle rub can do wonders. I have also listed some supplements that may help reduce postworkout discomfort and speed recovery. Supplements that are also listed in the Hot Hundred are designated by an asterisk.

Feed Your Hungry Muscles

ARGININE*. Arginine is an *amino acid*, a building block of protein. A recent study showed that arginine, along with carbohydrates, can enhance the release of insulin by the pancreas, resulting in a more rapid production of muscle glycogen. When combined with the amino acid ornithine, arginine can stimulate boost production of growth hormone, important to grow muscles and lose fat.

Do not use arginine if you have kidney or liver disease, unless under your doctor's supervision. Avoid arginine if you have herpes (either genital or oral), it can stimulate replication of the virus. Take three grams arginine after exercise, along with your carb snack.

BRANCHED-CHAIN AMINO ACIDS*. Branched-chain amino acids are three essential amino acids with special talents: leucine, isoleucine, and valine. Under normal circumstances, carbohydrates are burned as fuel but, during an intense workout, when you are placing unusual work demands on your body, protein may be broken down and burned as fuel. Due to their molecular structure, BCAAs are readily converted into glucose, which is converted to glycogen. BCAAs not only help to spare protein to build and repair muscles, but also enhance glycogen synthesis. Replenish your supply of BCAAs one hour before to one hour after working out.

GLUTAMINE*. *Glutamine* is another amino acid that helps replenish glycogen. It is also essential for the production of glutathione. Glutamine, which is also important for muscle repair, can reduce the amount of lactic acid in muscle after a difficult workout. Glutamine is available in powder, which is the most economical form. Mix one teaspoon glutamine in liquid. Drink up to one hour immediately before and immediately following your workout.

Restore Lost Antioxidants

LIPOIC ACID (ALPHA LIPOIC ACID)*. Lipoic acid can boost levels of glutathione while enhancing the effects of other key antioxidants vitamins C and E. It can help spare your body from the wear and tear of constant exposure to free radicals. Interestingly, lipoic acid is also instrumental in the production of ATP. After vigorous exercise, cells need extra energy for repair and recovery. If you don't have enough ATP, you cannot build new muscle. If you don't have enough lipoic acid, you will not have enough ATP. Take two 50 mg. tablets daily.

VITAMIN E*. Endurance and strength-training athletes need vitamin E supplements to prevent muscle damage due to free radicals. In one study of male college students, exhaustive exercise resulted in a sharp increase in serum lipid peroxide levels, a marker for free radicals, and elevated levels of key enzymes indicated free-radical muscle damage. When the men were given 300 IU of vitamin E for four weeks, the levels of free radicals dramatically decreased after exhaustive exercise, and enzyme activity was lower. In other words, vitamin E should help them retain muscle. Other studies have shown that athletes have significant skeletal muscle damage (as measured by levels of the intramuscular enzyme *creatine kinase*, a marker of cell damage) after a vigorous workout. However, when athletes take vitamin E, their levels of creatine kinase are much lower twenty-four hours after exercise than men taking a placebo! So, if you want to save your muscle, take 500 IU daily of the natural dry form of vitamin E.

WHEY PROTEIN POWDERS*. Here's a way to kill two birds with one stone—you can boost glutathione levels while, at the same time, enhancing your muscle strength. Whey, a high-quality protein derived from cow's milk, is a rich source of several amino acids, including the branched-chain amino acids needed to repair and build muscle. Studies show that whey protein can boost blood levels of glutathione, a critical antioxidant depleted during strenuous exercise. Mix two tablespoons daily in water. Take right before or after your workout.

10

PEAK PERFORMANCE TIPS ON PLAYING IT SAFE

Whether you're a student athlete or a weekend warrior, a sports injury—even a relatively minor one—can take you out of the game for weeks or months at a time. Not only can it prevent you from achieving your fitness goals, you can lose your momentum. There's always a risk that once you've stopped exercising regularly, you won't begin again.

Contrary to popular belief, athletic injuries are not an unfortunate fact of life. The reality is that most can be prevented. If they do occur, and are treated promptly, small problems need not escalate into larger ones.

Here's what you need to know to keep yourself and your kids out of harm's way.

Do You Have the Right Protective Gear?

If you are engaging in a sport in which you have the option of wearing protective gear, you should wear it. This sounds obvious yet, all too often, people don't bother using bike helmets, knee and elbow pads, protective goggles, and mouth guards that could prevent serious injury. Protective gear is particularly important for kids. Many states now require that children wear bike helmets but, drive along any suburban street and you'll see children (and adults) without them. In fact, a recent study showed that, out of 400,000 children treated for bike-related injuries, up to 45,000 head injuries could have been prevented if the children had only worn their helmets. In fact, about two-thirds of the injured children did have bike helmets. Make it a house rule that no one can go bicycle riding—including adults—without a helmet.

Head injuries are particularly common in softball and baseball, yet most kids and adults don't wear protective head gear or mouth pieces. In fact, many youth leagues don't require protective gear, even for catchers at home plate, who are not only at risk of being hit by the ball, but by being clobbered by the bat! Kids will not take the proper precaution on their own. It's up to parents and coaches to make the rules and to follow them.

Outdoor Protection

Most dermatologists believe that the leading cause of cancer is exposure to the sun's UV rays. In fact, the vast majority of skin problems (wrinkles, crow's feet, laugh lines) are due to photoaging. There are two types of ultraviolet rays: UVA and UVB. Both promote the formation of free radicals, which can turn healthy cells cancerous. UVB rays are the ones that actually burn your skin and make it red. UVA rays are not burning rays, but inflict significant damage underneath the top layers of skin. It's not just adults who need to worry about sun exposure. In reality, the damage begins early in life—it is cumulative and can take years before it is apparent. If you are engaged in an outdoor sport or activity on a regular basis, you need to take steps to protect your skin. Whenever possible, avoid spending time outdoors during the peak burning times, from 10 AM to 3 PM. Always wear a hat to protect your face, which is especially vulnerable to UV radiation. Never go out without using sunscreen of at least an SPF 15, which means that, if it normally takes a person fifteen minutes to burn, you can stay out in the sun fifteen times longer without burning. That doesn't give you license to bask in the sun for 150 minutes! Although you may not be burning, UVA rays are still causing damage to your skin. Look for a sunscreen that protects against both UVA and UVB rays. Reapply it often. (If you have sensitive skin, please test a sunscreen on a small patch of skin on your upper arm before using on your face and body.)

If you spend a lot of time in the sun, consider taking mixed carotenoids, a peak performance supplement (see page 47.) A recent study showed that natural mixed carotenoids can help protect skin against sun damage and reduce sensitivity to UV radiation. It appears to work well in combination with vitamin E. Take 60–90 mg. mixed carotenoids daily, with 400 IU of vitamin E.

Sun damage doesn't stop at your skin: It can cause cataracts and other eye problems. Be sure to wear UVA/UVB guard sunglasses when you are outdoors.

In some parts of the country, sun is not the only thing you have to worry about outdoors. In these areas, bug bites are not only unpleasant, but can be life threatening. By now everyone knows of the danger of Lyme disease, spread by deer ticks. There is now a new threat on the East Coast: West Nile virus, which is spread by mosquitos. Your best protection is to cover up! Wear long-sleeved shirts and long pants in heavily wooded areas. And do use a natural bug repellent. (Bite Blocker made from soybean oil is quite effective.)

Learning From Your Injury

There are two primary causes of athletic injuries—overtraining and undertraining. In both cases, the root of the problem is the same; you're pushing your body beyond its current limits.

OVERTRAINING. Overtraining is a more obvious problem. You're preparing for a marathon and you push harder and harder every day until, one day, you hurt so badly, you can't move. Or you're at the gym, and you're impatient with your rate of progress. So, you pick up your pace on the treadmill, or lift a heavier weight, and, then, ouch! You sprain an ankle, or your knee gives out, or you wrench your back. Your injury is a warning sign that you went too far and need to slow down. You also need to be better able to pick up early warning signs that your body is in trouble. Anyone who works out is going to have some degree of pain—lifting weights and stretching tight muscles can cause discomfort, to say the least. However, there are times when you must stop. Sharp pain is never normal. Swelling, particularly from joints, is a sign of injury. Feeling unusually sore after a workout is also a sign that you're overdoing it.

UNDERTRAINING. Undertraining is a more subtle problem, particularly for weekend athletes. You're chained to your desk during the week, but on Friday take off for a glorious weekend skiing the first snow of the season. Your first time on the slopes, you blow out your knee! Or, after months of being sedentary, you decide to play an aggressive game of basketball with some neighborhood kids. You slam dunk one too many times, and end up pulling your hamstring. That's it—you decide that you're too old for this stuff, and you better just give it up! Unfortunately, few weekend athletes learn the right lesson from their injury. The problem is that your muscles are getting weak. Instead of hanging up the towel, it's time to get yourself to a strength training class. The sudden increase in activity has revealed that your body is vulnerable. Your next injury may not occur on the slopes or the playing field, but could occur when you're running up a flight of steps or carrying a heavy package.

THE IMPORTANCE OF WARMING UP. If you injure easily, it could be a sign that you aren't warming up properly. Cold muscles are more likely to be injured, particularly as you get older. Whereas a fifteen-year-old athlete can warm up in five minutes, a fifty-year-old athlete needs at least fifteen to twenty minutes to get their muscles exercise ready.

How to Treat an Injury

Most minor injuries can be treated successfully at home. However, if you are in severe pain, if swelling persists for more than two days, or if things just don't feel right, call your doctor.

First, if something hurts, give it a rest. Don't exercise for a few days and avoid exerting the injured area. Second, apply ice to the injured area to reduce inflammation. (Be sure to wrap the ice in a washcloth to avoid direct contact with your skin.) Ice treatment is amazingly effective, as long as you don't overdo it. Use ice for only ten minutes at a time; if you keep it on longer, it can be irritating. Never apply heat to a fresh injury! It could increase swelling. If it helps, you can use a heating pad a day or two after the injury. Don't burn yourself—use only the lowest settings. Finally, keep the injured area elevated, particularly immediately following the injury. Rubs and ointments directly to the affected area may help reduce pain and inflammation. Creams containing capsaicin, boswellia, and eucalyptus are useful for sore muscles and joints.

By all means, start exercising again as soon as you can, but keep in mind that you may have to work around the sore area. Before resuming exercise, check with your doctor or a qualified physical trainer to make sure that you're not causing further damage.

What about painkillers, natural or otherwise? There are numerous over-the-counter NSAIDs (nonasteroidal anti-inflammatory drugs) used to treat pain and inflammation. They include aspirin, ibuprofen, and naproxen. On the plus side, they work fast and can relieve pain. On the minus side, they have some miserable side effects including gastrointestinal problems, ranging from upset stomach to bleeding ulcers. I prefer natural alternatives, but I must tell you that they take longer to work. If you must use an NSAID, I recommend that you do so sparingly, only when absolutely necessary. There are several excellent natural anti-inflammatories that will help promote the healing process. (Supplements that are also listed in the Hot Hundred are designated by an asterisk.)

BROMELAIN*. *Bromelain* is an enzyme derived from pineapple. It is a well-known anti-inflammatory. In fact, some studies have shown that bromelain is such an effective painkiller that it can reduce the need for corticosteroids in patients with severe arthritis. Keep in mind that bromelain isn't going to work overnight but, if you have an injury that keeps acting up, it could help reduce your discomfort over time. Take one 500 mg. capsule twice daily.

FLAVONOIDS*. Found in grapes, onions, red pepper, and citrus fruits, *flavonoids* are not only powerful antioxidants, but have been used successfully to treat bruises and muscles sprains. They work in synergy with vitamin C. Flavonoids helps reduce inflammation and strengthen cell membranes. According to a recent study conducted at San Jose College, flavonoid supplements and vitamin C reduced sport injuries by 50 percent and increased the rate of recovery from muscle injury by 50 percent. Interestingly, football players at Louisiana State University healed faster from muscle injuries when they took flavonoid supplements. I believe flavonoid supplements are a must for all athletes, amateur and pro alike, and they're even safe for teenagers. Take 1000 mg. mixed citrus flavonoids daily.

GLUCOSAMINE*. *Glucosamine* is a naturally occurring substance found in all human tissue, but in highest concentrations in *articular cartilage*, the thin coating that allows joints to move with fluidity. Glucosamine (along with chondroitin) is known as an arthritis cure. Glucosamine may also help promote the healing of overuse injuries. If you are recovering from an injury, I suggest that you try glucosamine—it may speed up your recovery. Many athletes swear by it. Take up to three 500 mg. tablets daily.

WHITE WILLOW*. Known as *natural aspirin*, the bark of the white willow tree is a natural source of *salicin*, the plant chemical that was synthesized into aspirin (acetylsalicylic acid) by German scientists in the 1850s. White willow, used to treat common body aches and pains, is also an anti-inflammatory. Over time, it could help relieve a chronically sore joint or muscle. Unlike aspirin, white willow contains tannins and flavonoids which could be soothing to the stomach. However, I still think it's wise for people with ulcers or an irritable gastrointestinal system to steer clear of both aspirin and white willow. Take 60–120 mg. standardized salicin extract for up to six weeks.

BIBLIOGRAPHY

Almada, A. "Three Experimental Biology Meeting Reports." *Nutrition Science News* (4) 9 (September 1999).

————. "Ergogenics 2000: Science-Based Performance Agents Are Fueling the Sports Industry." *Health Products Business* (May 2000).

Ames, B. N., et al. "Oxidants, Antioxidants and the Degenerative Diseases of Aging." Proceedings of the National Academy of Sciences of the United States of America 90:7915–22 (1993).

Arenas, J., et al. "Effects of L-Carnitine on the Pyruvate Dehyrogenase Complex and Carnitine Palmitoyl Transferase Activities in Muscle of Endurance Athletes." *FEBS Letters* 341:91–93 (1994).

Astrup, A., et al. "The Effect of Ephedrine/Caffeine Mixture on Energy Expenditure and Body Composition in Obese Women." *Metabolism* (41):686–688 (July 1992).

Bahrke, M., and W. Morgan. "Evaluation of Ergonomic Properties of Ginseng." *Sports Medicine* (18) 4: 229–248 (1994).

Balsom, P., et al. "Creatine Supplementation and Dynamic High Intensity Intermittent Exercise." *Scand Journal Med Sci Sports* (3) 143–149 (1993).

Bhattacharya, S. K., et al. "Effects of Glycowithanolides from Withania Somnifera on an Animal Model of Alzheimer's Diseae and Perturbed Central Cholinergic Markers of Cognition in Rats." *Phytotherapy Research* 9:110–113 (1995).

Blomstrand, E., et al. "Influence of Ingesting a Solution of Branched Chain Amino Acids on Perceived Exertion During Exercise." *Acta Physiol Scan* (159):41–49 (1997).

Braeckman, J. "The Extract of Sereno Repens in the Treatment of Benign Prostatic Hyperplasis: A Multicenter Open Study." *Current Therapy Research* 55:776–785 (1994).

Brewitt, B., et al. "Homeopathic Human Growth Hormone for Physiologic and Psychological Health." *Alternative & Complementary Therapies* (December 1999).

Brilla, L., and T. Haley. "Effect of Magnesium Supplementation on Strength Training in Humans." *Journal of the American College of Nutrition* (11)3:326–329 (1992).

Brown, R., et al. *Stop Depression Now: SAM-e, the Breakthrough Supplement That Works As Well As Prescription Drugs, in Half the Time . . . with No Side Effects.* New York: Penguin / Putnam, 1999.

Burke, Edmund. "A Critical Look at Androstenedione." *Nutrition Science News* (3) 11 (November 1998).

———. "OKG: Immunonutrient and Anabolic All in One." *Let's Live* (June 1999).

Cannon, J., et al. "Acute Phase Response in Exercise: Interaction of Age and Vitamin E on Neutraphils and Muscle Enzyme Release." *American Physiological Society* R1214-R1219 (1990).

Carotenoids Fact Book. La Grange, Ill. Veris Research Information Service, 1999.

Castell, L. M., and E. A. Newsholme. "Glutamine and the Effects of Exhaustive Exercise Upon the Immune Response." *Can J Physiol. Pharmacol* (76): 524–532 (1998).

Chandon, K., et al. "Oxidative Stress After Human Exercise: Effect of N-acetylcysteine Supplementation." *The American Physiological Society* (1994).

Christianson, A. "For the Road: Essential Nutrients for Athletes." *Nutrition Science News* (4)5:242–244 (May 1999).

Clark, D., and K. Wyatt. *Colostrum: Life's First Food, The Ultimate Anti-Aging, Weight Loss and Immune Supplement.* Salt Lake City: CNR Publications, 1996.

Coleston, D., and I. Hindmarch. "Possible Memory Enhancing Properties of Vinpocetine." *Drug Development Research* (14):191–193 (1988).

Cosgrove, J. "Cardiovascular Support." *Nutritional Outlook* (September 1999).

Cutler, W., et al. "Pheromonal Influences on Sociosexual Behavior in Men." *Archives of Sexual Behavior* (27)1 (1998).

Deal, C. L. "Treatment of Arthritis with Topical Capsaicin: A Double-Blind Trial." *Clinical Therapy* (13) 3:383–395 (May-June, 1991).

———. "DHEA Treatment for Sexual Dysfunction." *Life Extension* (January 2000).

Dulloo, A.G., and D. S. Miller. "Aspirin as a Promoter of Ephedrine-Induced Thermogenesis in the Obese." *American Journal of Clinical Nutrition* (45):3. 564–569 (March 1987).

Dulloo, A. G. "Efficacy of a Green Tea Extract Rich in Catechin Polyphenols and Caffeine in Increasing 24-Hour Energy Expenditure and Fat Oxidation in Humans." *American Journal of Clinical Nutrition* (70):1040–1045 (1999).

Elam, R. P. "Morphological Changes in Adult Males from Resistance Exercise and Amino Acid Supplementation." *Journal of Sports Medicine and Physical Fitness* 28: 35–39 (1988).

Firshein, R. *The Nutraceutical Revolution.* New York: Riverhead Books, 1998.

Gallaway, S. *The Steroid Bible: Third Edition.* Sacramento, CA: Belle International, 1997.

Germano, C., and Z. Ramazanov. *Arctic Root: The Powerful New Ginseng Alternative.* New York: Kensington Publishing Corp., 1999.

Germano, C. *The Osteoporosis Solution.* New York: Kensington Publishing Corp., 1999.

Gohil, K., et al. "Effect of Exercise Training on Tissue Vitamin E and Ubiquinone Content." *Journal of Applied Physiology* 63 (4) 1638–41 (1987).

Gormley, James. "Boswellia serrata: An Ancient Herb for Arthritis, Cholesterol and More." *Better Nutrition* (March 1996).

Grandhi, A., et al. "A Comparative Pharmacological Investigation of Ashwagandha and Ginseng." *J Ethnopharmacology* (44) 3: 131–135.

Hadady, L. "Chinese Herbs Enhance Sexual Vitality." *Nutrition Science News* (4)3:122 (March 1999).

Heymsfield, S. B., et al. "Garcinia Cambrogia (Hydrocitric Acid) as a Potential Antiobesity Ingredient." *Journal of the American Medical Association* (280) 1596–1600 (1998).

Hibblen, J. R., and M. Salem. "Dietary Polyunsaturated Fatty Acids and Depression." *American Journal of Clinical Nutrition* (62) 1:1–9.

Jacob, S., et al. *The Miracle of MSM: The Natural Solution for Pain.* New York: Penguin / Putnam, 1998.

Kaats, G., et al. "Effects of Chromium Picolinate Supplementation on Body Composition: A Randomized, Double-Masked, Placebo Controlled Study." *Current Therapeutic Reseach* (57)10:747–756 (October 1996).

Kantor, M. "Free Radicals, Exercise and Antioxidant Supplementation." *International Journal of Sport Nutrition* (4) 205–220 (1994).

Khalsa, K. P. S. "Peruvian Sex Herb and More . . . Maca." *Let's Live* (November, 1999).

Kilhan, C. "Maca: The Sex Plant of the Incas." *Total Health* (22)2.

King, D., et al. "Effect of Oral Androstenedione on Serum Testosterone and Adaptations to Resistance Training in Young Men." *Journal of the American Medical Association* (281) 21 (June 2, 1999).

Kinscherf, R., et al. "Low Plasma Glutamine in Combination with High Glutamate Levels Indicate a Risk for Loss of Body Cell Mass in Healthy Individuals: The Effect of N-acetyl cysteine." *J Mol Med* 74: 393–400 (1996).

Klatz, R., and R. Goldman. *Stopping the Clock.* New Canaan, CT: Keats Publishing, 1996.

Kreider, R. B., et al. "Effects of Creatine Supplementation During Training on the Incidence of Muscle Cramping, Injuries and GI Distress." *Journal of Strength and Conditioning Research* (12) 4: 275 (1998).

Le Bars, P. L., et al. "A Placebo-Controlled, Double-Blind, Randomized Trial of Extract of Ginkgo Biloba for Dementia." (North American EbG Study Group). *Journal of the American Medical Association* (278)1327–1332.

Liebelt, R. A., and D. Calcagnetti. "Effects of Bee Pollen Diet on the Growth of the Laboratory Rat." *American Bee Journal* 390–395 (May 1999).

Linsken, H. F., and W. Jorde. "Pollen as Food and Medicine: A Review." *Economic Botany* (51) 1 (1998).

Luppa, D., and H. Loster. "L-Carnitine Through Urine and Sweat in Athletes in Dependence on Energy Expenditure During Training." *Ponte Press Bochum* 278–279 (1996).

McAlindon, T., et al. "Glucosamine and Chondroitin for Treatment of Osteoarthritis: A Systematic Quality Assessment and Meta-Analysis." *Journal of the American Medical Association* (283) 11: 1469–1475 (March 15, 2000).

Maher, T. J. *Glucosamine Continuing Education*. Boulder, CO: New Hope Natural Media, 2000.

McCaleb, Rob. *What's New with Ginseng?* Herb Research Foundation. December 18, 1990.

Mooney, L. "Should You Decaf Your Life?" *Prevention* (July 2000).

Mindell, Earl. *Earl Mindell's Supplement Bible*. New York: Fireside, 1998.

———. *Earl Mindell's New Herb Bible*. New York: Fireside, 2000.

———. *Earl Mindell's Food as Medicine*. New York: Fireside, 1994.

———. *Earl Mindell's Vitamin Bible*. New York: Warner Books, 1999.

Naguib, Y., et al. "Nature's Super Antioxidant." *Total Health* (22) 4.

———. "New Study Confirms CLA's Anti-Fat Effects." *Life Extension* (February 2000).

———. NIDA Research Report. "Anabolic Steroids: A Threat to Body and Mind." Rockville, Md. (NIH Publication No. 96–3721.)

Nissen, S., et al. "Effect of Leucine Metabolite B-hydroxy-B-methylbutyrate on Muscle Metabolism During Resistance Exercise Training." *Journal of Applied Physiology* (81) 2095–2104 (1996).

Packer, L., and C. Colman. *The Antioxidant Miracle*. New York: John Wiley & Sons, 1999.

Passwater, R. "NADH: More Than an Energy Supplement." *Whole Foods Magazine* (April 1997).

———. *All About Selenium*. New York: Avery Publishing, 1999.

Pavlovic, P., et al. "Human Response to Physical-Stress Improved by Antioxidants." Abstract presented at the Oxygen Society Annual Meeting, Santa Barbara, CA, November 1998.

Pressman, A. *The GSH Phenomenon*. New York: St. Martin's Press, 1997.

Ramazanov, Z., and M. del Mar Bernal Suarez. *New Secrets of Effective Natural Stress and Weight Management Using Rhodiola Rosea and Rhododendron Caucasicum*. East Canaan, CT: ATN/Safe Goods Publishing, 1999.

———. "Replenish Testosterone Naturally." *Life Extension* (January 2000).

———. "Rev Up with Ribose." *Whole Foods* (March 2000).

Rice-Evans, C., and L. Packer. *Flavonoids in Health and Disease.* New York: Marcel Dekker, Inc., 1998.

Ryan, M. "Sports Drinks: Research Asks for Reevaluation of Current Recommendations." *Journal of the American Dietetic Association* (97)10. S197–198 (1997).

Sahelian, R., and D. Tuttle. *Creatine: Nature's Muscle Builder.* New York: Avery Publishing Group, 1997.

Simopoulos, A. P. "Omega-3 Fatty Acids in Health and Disease and in Growth and Development." *American Journal of Clinical Nutrition* (49)11:323–331 (1991).

Stanko, R.T., et al. "Body Composition, Energy Utilization, and Nitrogen Metabolism with a 4.25 MJ/d Low-Energy Diet Supplemented with Pyruvate." *American Journal of Clinical Nutrition* (56) 4: 630–635 (1992).

Subhan, Z., and I. Hindmarch. "Pharmacological Effects of Vinpocetine in Healthy, Normal Volunteers." *Eur J Clin Pharmacol* (28):567–571 (1985).

Suttie, J. "Role of Steroids in Antler Growth of Red Deer Stags." *Journal of Experimental Zoology* (221)2:12–130 (1995).

Teeguarden, R. *Chinese Tonic Herbs.* Tokyo: Japan Publications, 1984.

Thein, L.A., et al. "Ergonomic Aids." *Physical Therapy* 75(5):426–39 (1995).

Theodosakis, J., et al. *The Arthritis Cure.* New York: St. Martin's Press, 1997.

Toubro, S., et al. "Safety and Efficacy of Long-Term Treatment with Ephedrine, Caffeine and an Ephedrine/Caffeine Mixture." *International Journal of Obesity* (17) Suppl. 1: (S69–72) (1993).

Tuttle, D. "The Brain Nutrient That Protects Brawn." *Let's Live* (November 1997).

Ullis, K. *Super "T": The Complete Guide to Creating an Effective, Safe, and Natural Testosterone Enhancement Program for Men and Women.* New York: Fireside, 1999.

———. *Vitamin E Fact Book*. La Grange, IL: VERIS Research Information Service, 1999.

Ullman, R., and J. Reichenberg-Ullman. *Homeopathic Self-Care*. New York: Prima Publishing, 1997.

Walsh, D. E., et al. "Effect of Glucomannan on Obese Patients: A Clinical Study." *International Journal of Obesity* (8) 4:289–293 (1984).

Webb, S. "Do Weight Loss Supplements Ever Work?" *Prevention* (February 2000).

Werbach, M. "Sperm Count and Motility Improve with Nutrients." *Nutrition Science News* (3):12 (December 1998).

Whitaker, J., and C. Colman. *Shed 10 Years in 10 Weeks*. New York: Simon & Schuster, 1999.

Wu, Y. N., et al. "Effect of Cuwujia Preparation on Human Stamina." *Journal of Hygiene Research* (25) 1:57–61 (January 1996).

Zeligs, M. *All About DIM*. New York: Avery Publishing Group, 2000.

Zenk, J. *Living Longer in the Boomer Age*. Hauppauge, NY: Advanced Research Press, 1998.

Zhu, Xiao-Dong, and Xi Can Tang. "Improvement of Impaired Memory in Mice by Huperzine A and Huperzine B." *Acta Phamacologica. Sinica* (6):492–497 (1988).

INDEX

abdominal fat, reducing, 42
acetylcholine, 71, 126
acetylcholinesterase, 104, 215
aches, after exercise, 92, 233–34, 240
  see also soreness, after exercise
adaptogens, 27, 85
adenonine nucleotides, 138
adenosine triphosphate, *see* ATP
adenylate cyclase, 81
adolescents, *see* teenagers
adrenal glands, 129, 161
advanced glycation end products
  (AGEs), 115
aerobic exercise, 26, 219
age spots, 115
aging, 26, 32, 93, 164
  bone loss and, 218; *see also*
    osteoporosis
  brain function and, 35, 84, 85,
    210–12, 214, 215
  DHEA levels and, 66
  memory loss and, 71–72
  mitochondria and, 227
  muscle loss and, 217–18
  reversing process of, 60, 61,
    106–7, 228–29
  skin and, 47, 48, 115, 238
  stress and, 212
  testosterone level and, 150
Agriculture Department, U.S.,
  (USDA), 132
AIDS, 62, 101
alanine, 22, 175
alcohol, 95, 124, 160, 209, 213
  sex life and, 201
  teenagers and, 194
alcoholism, 75
allergies, 37, 80, 81

alpha ketaglutate, 124–25
alpha linolenic acid, 182
alpha-2 receptors, 168–69
*Alternative and Complementary
  Therapy*, 103
Alzheimer's disease, 25, 27, 33, 65,
  71, 72, 84, 119, 124, 153, 159,
  212, 215, 216
American ginseng, 86
American Heart Association, 142
American Journal of Clinical Nutrition,
  48
amino acids, 94, 117, 175, 198
  arginine, 29–30, 101, 107, 125,
    126, 143, 203–4, 234
  branched-chain (BCAAs), 40–42,
    165, 198, 213, 234–35
  creatine, 62–64, 101, 119, 197–98,
    230
  defined, 40
  essential, nonessential, and
    conditionally essential, 175
  glutamine, 91–93, 101, 124, 143,
    235
  leucine, 41, 100, 114, 175, 213,
    222, 234
  methionine, 45, 119–20, 153,
    175
  OKG, 124–25
  ornithine, 29, 125–26, 234,
    125–26
  tyrosine, 154–55, 214
amphetamines, 212
anabolic action, 16
anabolic steroids, 212
  andro compared to, 23, 24
  side effects of, 196
  teenagers and, 195–97

About the Author

Earl Mindell, R.Ph., Ph.D., is the bestselling author of *Earl Mindell's Vitamin Bible* in addition to *Earl Mindell's New Herb Bible*, *Earl Mindell's Supplement Bible*, *Earl Mindell's Secret Remedies*, *Earl Mindell's Anti-Aging Bible*, *Earl Mindell's Soy Miracle*, and *Earl Mindell's Food as Medicine*. He is a registered pharmacist, a master herbalist, and a professor of nutrition at Pacific Western University in Los Angeles; he also conducts nutrition seminars around the world. He lives in Beverly Hills, California.